A DOCTOR IN THE WILDERNESS

A DOCTOR IN THE WILDERNESS

Walter W. Yellowlees

JANUS PUBLISHING COMPANY
London, England

First published in Great Britain 1993
by Janus Publishing Company
Duke House, 37 Duke Street, London W1M 5DF

British Library Cataloguing-in-Publication Data.
A catalogue record for this book is available
from the British Library.

ISBN 1 85756 013 2

Cover design Linda Wade

Printed & bound in England by
Antony Rowe Ltd, Chippenham, Wiltshire

To Sonia, Robin, Michael and Jane

Contents

List of figures	9
List of tables	11
Foreword by Professor N. J. Blacklock	13
Acknowledgements	15
Introduction	17
Chapter 1 Partnerships	21
2 Trouble in the Glen	27
3 Childbirth	31
4 Convertible Births	39
5 Work, Leisure and Fatigue	42
6 Varicose Veins	51
7 Surgeon-Captain T. L. Cleave	55
8 Maggie and her Constipation	66
9 A Case of Cancer	73
10 More on Cancer	80
11 Scurvy on the Farm	87
12 Simple Causes	92
13 Birth in a Tent	95
14 Angus, Jock and their Insulin	101
15 Overconsumption	106
16 Duodenal Ulcer, Stress and Food-Combining	114
17 Rheumatism, Homeopathy: Physician Heal Thyself	123
18 A ken fine it's his appendix	128
19 The Scourge of Coronary Thrombosis	139
20 Coronary Thrombosis: Fats Ancient and Modern	145
21 Cholesterol and The Censorship of Fashion	155
22 Remembrance: Battles Long Ago	167
23 Remembrance: Decline and Fall	177
24 Remembrance: Land and People	184
25 Hell on Earth	195
Epilogue	204
Appendixes 1 Advice to consumers	207
2 Advice to Government	219
Index	225

Figures

Fig. 1 Aberfeldy practice, visits and consultations 1962–80   22
      2 All types of malformation by social class   35
      3 Industrial extraction of sugar from parent plant   57
      4 Alteration of wheat by milling   58
      5 Composition of English flours   59
      6 Diseases caused by eating refined carbohydrates   62
      7 Household food consumption   76
      8 Percentage of persons aged 44 years who will *not* survive
        to age 65 years in Sweden and in the UK   78
      9 Deaths from spina bifida in first year   98
     10 Operations for appendicitis in Edinburgh Royal Infirmary
                                                                 131
     11 Rise in sugar consumption in the UK 1800–1960   133
     12 T. L. Cleave's incubation period fuse   137

Tables

Table 1: Effect of dietary fibre on stools and transit times   69

2: Purchase of butter, margarine and spreads   147

3: Fat supplies and death rates in certain European countries and USA   151

4: Consumption of centrifugal sugar by countries, pre-war average and 1958   153

5: Sugar consumption by UK and Japan   153

6: Daily per caput intake and percentage of calories derived from protein, carbohydrate and fat   163

Foreword

By Professor N. J. Blacklock, CVO, OBE, Department of Urology, University Hospital of South Manchester

I have enjoyed reading this fascinating account of events in the life of a general practitioner in such an agreeable location in rural Scotland. Others will enjoy this book just as I did because of the way in which the author brings out that most important requirement for successful medical practice – and indeed the practice of medicine in general: an intimate knowledge of the patient as a person in his or her family surroundings. Reading this book will bring to some perhaps their first realisation of the art that is medicine, which is after all practised in its most pure form 'in general' and in a rural setting. The author has recounted a particularly important phase in the evolution of medical practice, beginning at a time when facilities and our ability significantly to affect the natural course of disease were much more restricted than they are now. In the course of his and our generation there have been monumental strides in medical progress. This has inevitably had its impact upon the practice in which he worked: nevertheless the 'basics' for good medicine remain as he has described them in this book.

Quite apart from the medical aspects which are inseparable from the text, Dr Yellowlees has provided us with something equally valuable. This is the description of the attitudes to life and the deep philosophy of the people with whom he was involved and the basic reality of the closeness to nature which is the lot of those living and working in rural surroundings. While some may still consider the rural setting to be a disadvantage, I believe an increasing number of people in towns and cities will greatly envy what he describes in these chapters as perhaps the life style which provides not only the potential for better health but for peace and contentment of mind as well.

Dr Yellowlees neatly combines within this book an important facet of his own medical ethos – his beliefs in the importance of healthy nutrition. As a past president of the society which has embraced this for many years – the McCarrison Society – Dr Yellowlees propounds within his book clinical examples which vividly illustrate the various tenets of these beliefs and their application both in the diagnosis of the disease and the management of the malady. I think his various anecdotes are well chosen and illustrative. He and I do not agree in every one of his beliefs but there is no denying the broad truth of the lesson he teaches. Happily, of recent weeks there has been acknowledgement by government of the further steps which we need to take in observing a dietary style which, while giving us adequacy of nutrition, will nevertheless not be harmful in excesses of such things as sugars and deficiency of whole cereal intake. He refers to other accounts of the health of the Highlander of yesteryear and laments the influence of the encroachment of the fast food and prepacked food industry on his practice. This pattern is repeated worldwide and it is to be hoped the communities less 'well developed' than ours at present will not be persuaded to follow the bad examples set by ourselves here in western Europe, North America and Australasia wherein are now so many of the diseases of so-called Western 'progress'.

I wish this book well. It deserves a wide readership for the solace, comfort and enlightenment it can provide from this account of a life well spent in rural general practice in Scotland.

Acknowledgements

The views expressed in this book are the result of contacts with so many people that to name them all would be impossible.

But for meeting the late Surgeon-Captain T. L. Cleave and his wife, Helen, I would not have attempted to write a book at all. Nor might I have persisted in the almost impossible task of trying to interpret the work of Cleave and McCarrison for both lay and medically qualified readers without the enthusiastic support of Peter Brown, BDS, LDS, RCS, of Guernsey, who shares my admiration for Cleave's teaching.

Another source of encouragement came from the outstanding educational work of Dr Kenneth Vickery, former MOH of the County Borough of Eastbourne.

Mrs Doris Grant, a staunch and long-standing ally, has been generous in giving me advice from her long experience as an author and researcher on many aspects of nutrition and health.

I am grateful for discussions over the years with members of the McCarrison Society – too numerous to mention by name. I crave their forgiveness for not mentioning them all, but wish to record that the survival and growth of the society in the 1970s and 80s was due to the dedication of the then secretary, Dr Barbara Latto and her husband, Gordon, through whom I met many distinguished nutritionists; and I must thank Margaret and Arthur Wynn for permission to use their valuable material on the incidence of congenital handicap.

On agriculture, much valuable information has been given to me by my brother Dave, of Muirhall Farm, Perth, by Jock Scott-Park of Gartocharn, by Tom Stockdale from Dumfriesshire, and more recently by Ian Millar whose organic farm, Jamesfield, in Fife, is now a focus of officially financed research into biological farming.

Membership of the Soil Association and my meeting with the late Lady Eve Balfour some forty years ago introduced me for the first time to all that is implied by the word 'ecology'; Lady Eve's example remains a constant source of inspiration. Of SA members, Jimmy Anderson has always cheerfully answered my horticultural queries.

On retiring from his post as consultant psychiatrist at Murray Royal Hospital in Perth, Dr Harry Stalker became an invaluable (unpaid!) research assistant to me; as part-time hospital librarian he kept me supplied with cuttings from medical and lay press on every conceivable aspect of nutrition and health.

My thanks are due to Dr Robin Hull for agreeing to read the first draft of the book and for his frank criticism, and to Campbell and Maisie Steven who also read the script and offered comments. Occasionally, when my woeful lack of skill in manipulating a wordprocessor landed me deep in trouble, either Roger Sylvester or Joe Gallacher promptly answered my distress calls. I record my gratitude for this invaluable help.

I am deeply grateful to Professor Norman Blacklock of the University Hospital of South Manchester for so generously giving his precious time to write a foreword.

Finally I wish to thank my former patients and friends who taught me so much and my wife, Sonia, for repeatedly and cheerfully undertaking the tedious task of correcting the script and for her suggestions and constant support.

Introduction

Wilderness. 'A region uncultivated and uninhabited: a pathless and desolate tract: . . . conditions of life, or a place in which the spirit feels desolate: . . . the present world: . . . a large confused or confusing assemblage' (*Chambers Twentieth Century Dictionary*).

Forty years ago, in April 1948, as I started on my morning round, I often waved to a tall white-haired man, walking, shepherd's crook in hand, on the Strathtay road. He was the late Dr Douglas MacKay who had recently retired from the Aberfeldy practice; I was then the newly arrived young doctor – curious, eager and a bit fearful as I plunged into the turmoil of the daily round.

As he walked up the strath, Dr MacKay no doubt pondered on the final chapters of his book, *Aberfeldy Past and Present,*[1] in which he was to record a mass of fascinating information about the people who lived in and around this small market town standing in the midst of the Perthshire Highlands.

Last year, on my seventieth birthday, my nephew gave me a beautiful shepherd's crook; so now, in my turn, I am the white-haired old doctor walking the dog, crook in hand. Ideas for a book have often been in my mind during the seven years since I retired from the practice in 1981; now that I have passed threescore years and ten, I realise that if I am to write a book I had better start now, before I, too, become the 'late' doctor. My book could not match Dr MacKay's grasp of local history, but the changes in medical practice and in the way of life of this community, once based on farming, have been so far-reaching in the last forty years, that I wanted to record the atmosphere of rural practice in the years immediately following Hitler's war.

My book, however, is not mainly concerned with developments in

1. N. D. MacKay, *Aberfeldy Past and Present* (Perthshire, Cupar Angus, Wm. Culross & Son, Abereldy, January 1988, 1953)

medical practice, interesting as they are; if a GP lives up to the traditions of his calling, he must for ever seek to understand why this particular patient is suffering from this particular complaint. When confronted with the baffling challenge of serious illness, doctors may assume two attitudes; the first views the illness as an unfortunate happening, a haphazard quirk of fate, which gives the doctor an opportunity of exercising his diagnostic and therapeutic skills; that is, after all, what he was trained for. The second attitude takes a much wider view which encompasses not only the patient's disease, but his way of life, food, relationships and environment. The latter attitude, in the Hippocratic tradition, assumes that health is the normal inheritance of mankind and seeks to know what has gone wrong to disturb that inheritance.

During the twentieth century, thanks to better sanitation, clean water, preventive inoculation and improved housing, the incidence of infective diseases caused by bacteria or viruses has greatly diminished. But illness due to non-infective, or degenerative, disease has dramatically increased; the rising tide, during the century, of afflictions such as appendicitis, duodenal ulcer, diabetes, gall stones, coronary thrombosis and other serious conditions including some forms of cancer, cannot, in my opinion, be explained as the consequence of better methods of diagnosis or the ageing of the population.

Prevention is now being urgently advocated by politicians, increasingly alarmed at the escalating costs of medical care; unfortunately, the widely agreed measures (improved sanitation and so on) for prevention of infection are not matched by similar agreement on the measures to prevent degeneration. Four lectures, which I published in a small booklet in 1985,[2] did not do justice to a subject of such vital importance. I have therefore attempted to enlarge on my theme by including individual cases as they occur in a rural setting.

Given a clean environment, I believe that of all factors which make for human health, the greatest single factor is sound nutrition, or to use McCarrison's phrase, 'perfectly constituted food'. In support of my belief in the simple dietary causes of modern diseases, I shall refer repeatedly to the work of the late Sir Robert McCarrison[3] and the late Surgeon-Captain T. L. Cleave;[4] I hope that critics who may be tempted to dismiss my views as nonsense will, at least, study the findings of these two distinguished scientists.

2. W. W. Yellowlees, *Food and Health in the Scottish Highlands* (Aberfeldy, Clunie Press, 1985)
3. Sir R. McCarrison, *Nutrition and Health* (London, Faber, 1953)
4. T. L. Cleave, *The Saccharine Disease* (Bristol, John Wright, 1974)

Introduction

General practitioners encounter diseases not as graphs or statistics but as suffering individuals; in rural practice they are often seen more as friends than as patients. In this setting, disease is viewed in a different light altogether from that which illuminates the researches of a scientist in laboratory or library. My study of disease processes has always been initiated by a wish to know why this man or woman whom I know so well should be afflicted by this particular disease.

A writer as academically humble as this one, who scans the literature of research into the dietary causes of modern degenerative disease, finds himself in a confusing wilderness of fierce claim and counter-claim. Results published by one group of scientists are sooner or later contradicted by another group. Food manufacturers, equipped with their immensely powerful weapons of mass advertising, join the fray; they do so either openly to the consumer or through a more subtle approach to doctors and dieticians by financing research, publications, or conferences.

But it is beyond the power of scientific method to assess over the long term the effects on human health of any particular dietary regime; people cannot, like laboratory animals, be caged, fed and observed over several generations; a multitude of environmental variables cannot be controlled, so all conclusions from dietary research are part guesswork. Dietary fashion, swayed by the evangelism of specialists and the power of commerce, is for ever changing. Today's dietary villain becomes tomorrow's hero.

The wilderness of dietary controversy is one aspect of my title; but like Caesar's Gaul it is divided into three parts. The second part is the majestic background of hill, moor and glen against which as a generalist I have been privileged to work and to draw my own conclusions about the causes and prevention of degenerative disease. My material is, of course, anecdote rather than science, and will be dismissed by most scientists as of no consequence. But if guesswork plays such a large part in our search for dietary truth, I wonder if a relatively isolated rural practice is not as good a place as any for making a reasonable guess. Is there a better way of knowing what this sick person eats than by visiting him or her at meal times? I live on the edge of the second wilderness and will tell a little of the struggle my wife and I waged to tame a small patch of it in order to grow our fruits and vegetables.

The third and daunting part of my wilderness is the spiritual darkness which, in the second half of this century, has cast a deepening shadow over all our affairs. By darkness I mean the loss of loyalty,

19

honesty, integrity and decency without which human transactions revert to the violence and inhumanity of the beast. These sad trends follow the retreat of Christianity and the rise of humanist false prophets who preach the supremacy not of God, but of human reason; they seek to rule the world, not by God-given wisdom, but by the power of money. In my closing chapters I will try and explore these things.

Warfare, however justified, is perhaps the darkest area of our spiritual wilderness; doctors enjoy a special privilege in being able to observe war at close quarters and still to practise their profession while doing so; I have therefore included one chapter in which I have tried to give a very personal experience of the wilderness of war.

One difficulty facing a GP who attempts to write a book such as this is the fear of betraying that trust and confidentiality which is such a precious thing in the doctor-patient relationship. Most of the clinical incidents here recorded happened more than twenty-five years ago. Some were published in the *Bulletin of the East of Scotland Faculty of the Royal College of General Practitioners*; I am grateful to the Faculty for allowing me to use the material. Alterations in names and places have been made in the hope of avoiding identification.

Aberfeldy, January 1988

1 Partnerships

The changes in farming practice in the upper Tay valley are part of a worldwide revolution which has been gathering pace since the early decades of the twentieth century. Mixed farming – the partnership of stock rearing with a strict rotation of varied crops – all with a view to maintaining and improving soil fertility, has now virtually disappeared.

The scatter of small family farms, whose tenants in 1948 cultivated the arable land of this valley, were able to continue these traditional methods in the 1950s before economic forces swept them away; in a few farms, horses were still used and farm bothies occupied. The farming community in the fifties was thus a considerable population which included many families with small children requiring medical care from the doctors based in Aberfeldy. There were ten primary schools within the practice boundary, which extends westwards some fifteen miles upriver from Aberfeldy to march with the Killin practice halfway along the shores of Loch Tay, and which includes in its westward half the strath of Appin, Kenmore, Fortingall and all of Glen Lyon. Downriver, east of Aberfeldy, the practice boundary includes the villages of Strathtay, Grandtully, Balnaguard and part of Ballinluig.

Today all the smaller farms have been merged into large units. Mixed farming is being replaced by specialisation and, here and there, by a kind of monoculture totally dependent on heavy applications of nitrogenous fertilisers. Ever more ingenious machines have taken over from manual labour; most of the small-farm families and their workers have gone. The number of primary schools in the practice area has been halved. The wider implications of the loss of rural populations and of changing techniques in agriculture are of profound worldwide importance. The flow of people from countryside to cities in time brings such congestion to the latter that they become uninhabitable. The partnership between man and the land which sustains him is

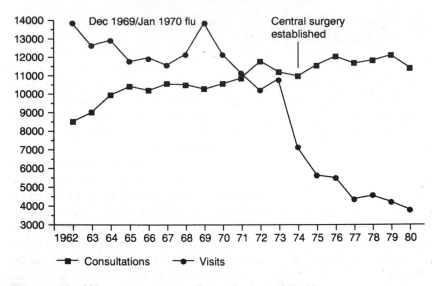

Fig. 1: *Aberfeldy practice, visits and consultations 1962–80*
(Source: author)

strained or broken. New generations of city-dwellers in their concrete jungles become ever more divorced from the great realities of the changing seasons, and from the use of land for sowing and reaping and rearing stock.

In the 1950s car ownership among the practice population was not nearly so widespread as now; the journey into the doctor's consulting room, especially for mothers with young children, was difficult; so we did far more visits than surgery consultations. Visiting the patient's home was maybe encouraged by the fact that, in the days before separate practice premises, the consulting room was usually a ground-floor room of the doctor's own house. There simply was not space for a crowd of patients in the hall or dining room; the receptionist was often the doctor's wife.

Fig. 1 shows the dramatic fall in the number of home visits, following the setting up in 1973 of a central practice consulting room and its appointment system; the change is a clear demonstration of how patterns of work in general practice can be determined more by a doctor's habits and organisation than by levels of ill-health.

Daily routine

In Aberfeldy the formal day's work began with a nine o'clock conference of partners, held for the purpose of arranging the day's visits. This took place at the house of the new senior partner, Dr Jack Swanson, to whom in 1947 I had applied as a possible successor to Dr Douglas MacKay. Jack Swanson was such a remarkable character that he deserves a separate biography. A man of immense strength and vigour, his capacity for work was astonishing; he appeared not to experience fatigue and required far less sleep than ordinary mortals like me. He was an entertaining conversationalist with an appropriate joke for every occasion and his patients adored him.

He had a prodigious memory, was an accomplished and witty speaker and had a unique grasp of the administration of the Highlands and Islands medical service, a system of state support for rural medical practice in the Highland area of Scotland which had been successfully running for many years before the advent of the National Health Service in 1948. His experience as a representative of rural practitioners for the Highlands and Islands service made him an obvious choice as a representative on the key Scottish committees of the new NHS. He relished medical politics, and his ability as a chairman gave him an important role to play in the unending negotiations which inevitably follow when the state takes over such a vast and complex service as the delivery of medical care. Within a few years of the establishment of the NHS, Jack's services on various committees of the British Medical Association were in such demand that he had to visit London at least once a month, sometimes more often.

His routine for London visits went something like this: in the days before the Forth road bridge he would rise at about 5 a.m., drive to Edinburgh airport to catch the London flight, then do his committee work all morning and most of the afternoon, usually at the British Medical Association headquarters or at the Department of Health. A late afternoon flight would return him to Edinburgh, and after the long 75-mile drive back to Aberfeldy he would arrive in time for supper at about 7.30 p.m. He would then go out to do a few home visits to patients, and from about 9.30 p.m until 1 a.m. or thereabouts would deal with his letters. The next morning he would be up early to wash his car before breakfast, a routine which he seldom failed to carry out. There was always the chance that his night would be disturbed by an emergency call. Even if he was so disturbed, the toil of the previous day seemed to leave him fresh and unruffled.

Between his London visits there were frequent journeys to Edinburgh, Perth, Glasgow or elsewhere and by the 1960s he was usually away from the practice for two or three days every week. His achievements, in the real sense of the word, were incredible. He was held in high regard both by the colleagues with whom he shared committee work and by the government officials. He won high honours, including the OBE in 1963, and in 1973 before retiring he was made a Vice-President of the British Medical Association, an honour reserved for those who have served the Association with great distinction.

In order to ease the practice work load, in 1951 we engaged the first of a series of annual assistants. This arrangement lasted until 1959 when a third partner in the person of Dr Ann Thomson of Dundee was invited to join the practice. Her presence and skill greatly enhanced the value of the partnership. There are always patients who prefer to consult a woman doctor.

To return to the 9 a.m. conference: arranging a day's visits had to be done with considerable care. On Mondays, Wednesdays and Fridays we visited eastwards, downriver; on Tuesdays, Thursdays and Saturdays westwards, upriver. This pattern was known throughout the practice, and patients were encouraged to keep their complaints (unless urgent!) to the appropriate day.

The morning conference lasted about thirty minutes and was useful for discussing clinical and other practice problems. Having drawn up our visiting lists and decided our various journeys, we would hurry to visit, first in the town and then in the cottage hospital. Coffee, presided over by Matron Jessie Cameron, was available at the hospital from 10 a.m. onwards; the danger of this was the temptation to sit blethering and so delay our departure for country visits. They had to be done in time to get back for a quick lunch before the consulting room session at 2 p.m. The afternoon consulting varied greatly in duration – possibly up to one and a half hours, after which there were usually more town or country visits or minor surgery at the hospital. Evening consulting started at 6.30 p.m and might go on until about 8 p.m.

Emergencies

Emergency calls often disrupt the best-laid schemes, especially in a rural practice with its own cottage hospital, where every accident or emergency must be dealt with by one of the local doctors. This is quite different from general practice in the city where most emergencies are dealt with by the hospital or ambulance service without the GP being troubled. Different also from the city practice is the annual pattern of work load. In the peak holiday months, as guest-houses, hotels, camp and caravan sites fill up with holidaymakers from the city, the rural work load increases; July and August can be as busy as winter.

Responsibility for all emergencies necessitates a system of communication by which at any time in the twenty-four hours one of the doctors can be located speedily. Modern radio telephones have partly solved this problem, but before their invention a somewhat primitive 'bush telegraph' had been evolved in Aberfeldy which worked remarkably well. Most of the outlying villages had, in those days, their own post office; a telegram envelope, stuck in the post office window, was a sign to the passing doctor that he must phone back to base, that is, his wife. This system required two items of daily drill, not to be forgotten – always tell your wife exactly where you are going and never pass a post office without looking at the window!

A biscuit box with a broom handle stuck in it, placed at the Strathtay road junction by the Gushat Store was another signal for the passing doctor to call at the store where the late Cyril Hunter kindly collected messages and passed them on. No thought, as far as I know, was ever given to the desirability of some form of reward to the post offices or to the store for these services. At a time when money did not seem to loom quite so large in all our affairs as it does now, the emergency-message network was accepted as part of an informal community service.

Another example of willing help in the practice was the hand-operated Aberfeldy telephone exchange. The splendid couple, Mr and Mrs Campbell, who manned the switchboard in their flat above the post office out of working hours, cheerfully took messages on the whereabouts of the doctor, and equally cheerfully called us at the cinema or town hall or the house of the friend whose telephone number we had left with them before going out. Stories abound about rural hand-operated telephone exchanges; our pair had an extraordinary knack of knowing where we were, even if we had forgotten to tell where we were going!

The key person in the communication system was the doctor's wife I lived with the Swansons for six months before I found and bought my own house, Inzievar, at the crossroads, and I soon came to appreciate and admire the devotion with which Jack's wife, Margaret, ran the household and acted as her husband's back-up, receptionist and sometimes secretary. She was a charming person, a marvellous cook and hostess; Jack's total absorption in the practice and in politics and his frequent absences must at times have made life difficult for her. So it was with doctors' wives in the 'bad old days'. I was fortunate when, in 1950, my wife Sonia came from distant Surrey and accepted the tyranny of the telephone and the doorbell, and the restriction these placed on her movements. As doctors of a past generation became more and more involved in the drama and responsibilities of general practice, they probably did not fully realise the adjustment that their wives had to make in accepting this strange life style.

In the days before full-time secretaries in general practice, daily help or living-in help was essential if the doctor's wife was not to be a prisoner in her own home. Without help it would have been impossible to survive the years when young children add to the chaotic workload of a GP household. Breakfast time could be particularly difficult – children eating (or refusing) breakfast and having to be got ready for school; the telephone shrilling incessantly, with demands for visits; or the front-door bell ringing to reveal a messenger or patient holding a bottle of urine for testing, or requesting the repeat of a prescription; occasionally a figure at the door grasping a bleeding limb, fresh from the scene of injury and requiring immediate care.

The 1965 reform of the system of paying GPs which enabled them to employ staff and to afford purpose-built premises, removed a doctor's wife and home from the day-to-day running of patient care. I am sure that overall the move to staffed premises has led to improvement in the standards of care in general practice, but centralised premises, especially for large groups of doctors, are apt to hinder the personal care which is such a precious thing in general practice.

2 Trouble in the Glen

As the following diary entry reveals, our practice communication network occasionally failed.

July 1951. The park, fringed by its trees and framed by the hills, was a carpet of green in the evening sun. The strip in the middle had been cut, rolled and marked; the wickets were standing ready and, the visiting team having arrived, players, some in white flannels, some dressed more informally, were casually practising with bat and ball beside the small pavilion. Of all Anglo-Saxon contributions to the gaiety of nations none must surely be more precious than the village cricket match. It gives scope for aggression without hate, and for skill and agility without too much of either; it has no barriers of class or age; in the same team, the aged laird can take his place with the budding schoolboy.

With these profound thoughts I had got out of my car and was strolling to the pavilion when the lady in the house bordering the park, who had a telephone, came running to say that I was wanted urgently. My wife, at the other end of the line, told me that a call had just come in from Glenlyon Post Office asking for a doctor to go at once to Tulloch farm where a shepherd was bleeding badly from a severe injury of his jaw. So I gave my apologies to our captain and rushed home.

The Glenlyon district nurse could not be contacted, so there seemed to be no alternative but to set out immediately. I had not been in the practice for long and this sounded to be an ugly situation. The problem of distance in rural practice is one which our urban colleagues often do not comprehend. Tulloch farm was thirty miles away, so the task facing me was as if a doctor practising, say, in Edinburgh, had to set out on an evening visit to a patient in Galashiels, or as if a Glasgow practitioner had to do the same for a

27

patient in Perth, with the difference that the main roads between these places are infinitely better than the one which winds its way up Glenlyon.

I checked my bag for dressings, artery forceps, sutures, and loaded in the car a couple of bottles of plasma. If this man was as badly injured as the message indicated why had they not put him in a vehicle and brought him forthwith to the Cottage Hospital? The journey takes an hour. Tulloch farm lies against the hills on the other side of the river. There being no bridge you can reach it either by a shallow ford which, if the water is not high, can be crossed by a tractor or horse and cart, or by the rowing boat kept chained by the bank of a long deep pool. If the boat is on the far side you give warning of your approach by a blast on the car horn, hoping that someone will come and ferry you across.

This evening the boat was at the nearside of the bank and either from the recent rain or from a leaky hull was deeply awash with water. The blade from one of the oars had broken off and was now held in place with a rough wooden splint secured by a couple of rusty nails reinforced by binder twine. In this emergency there was not time, I thought, to bail her so I took my seat and pushed off, keeping my feet as dry as I could by resting them on the gunwales.

Anyone who has tried to row a boat in this position will know that it is not a very good posture for efficient propulsion. But maybe it was just as well not to pull too hard, for if the starboard blade came adrift from its splint, I had fears, as I looked at the dark swirling water, of spinning out of control to humiliating wreckage on the rapids at the tail-end of the pool.

In cases of desperate urgency, such as I supposed this to be, there is usually someone on the lookout for the arrival of the doctor, but the two fields separating the farm from the river were deserted as I traversed them with haste sweating under the load of my two emergency bags. The fank behind the farm was loud with the noise of sheep and dogs, for clipping was in progress and the hill park was dotted with protesting, newly-shorn ewes, their shaved backs unusually white against the green grass. Mrs MacDonald opened the door.

'Oh! It's you doctor. We didn't expect you so soon.'

'The injured man,' I said, 'how is he?'

'Och, Willie, he's better now, just come through.'

In a small back room Willie, a shepherd I did not know, was lying on top of a bed. His countenance could hardly have looked less troubled; it was glowing with health and sunburn. He held a handkerchief, slightly bloodstained, and controlling my emotions with difficulty I discovered what had happened. Willie had been bending over a sheep working away with the clippers when he had a sharp nose-bleed. The bleeding had persisted so he had come to lie down; now it had stopped, that was all.

'You'll have a cup of tea, Doctor?'

An impulse to turn haughtily on my heel and sweep out, slamming the door, lasted only a moment. It is somehow difficult to be angry in the Glen. So I sat down meekly for my tea, which was indeed very welcome.

'Escalation' is now a fashionable word which best explains what happens to messages for the doctor in these parts. I never got the full details of how this message escalated, but after chatting over the teacups with Mrs MacDonald it seemed to have gone something like this. Willie's nose starts to bleed, so he goes and sits down. Still it bleeds and someone, pausing at his work with the sheep, says, 'Now I wonder if the doctor's in the Glen?'

Mr MacDonald, the head shepherd, feeling maybe that some action from him is called for, shouts to his ten-year-old son who is playing in the corner of the fank: 'Neil, go you down to the river and ask Mr Macpherson the keeper there on his bicycle if the doctor's about.'

So Neil runs to the river and shouts to Mr Macpherson, 'They want the doctor for Willie.'

'What's the matter with him?' replies Macpherson.

'Och, he's all blood about the mouth,' said Neil, for this is what he has seen.

A few moments later Mr Macpherson is overtaken by the grocer's van on its way home from the day's round and waves it to stop.

'Donald,' he says to the driver, 'tell them down at the Post Office to phone for the doctor; Willie up there at the Tulloch has had a bad accident and hurt his mouth. He's bleeding bad.'

Notice that the situation has now got beyond the point of no return. By this time Willie's nose has in fact stopped bleeding, but the team at the fank are so eager to finish their last batch of ewes that they have forgotten all about him and the call for a doctor. Ten miles downriver Donald's message to Jeanie the postmistress is for her a welcome break in the tedium of trying to make her day's cash balance. Serious illness, accidents and emergencies are for her like rays of sunshine in a cloudy evening. So she sets the wires humming and my wife, eager to do her best, takes down the details: a bad accident at Tulloch farm, losing blood from a broken jaw, doctor to come at once. . .

Neil carried my bags to the river and I was ferried across to the car. The keyline in this evening's farce was 'the District Nurse could not be contacted'. In scattered communities the District Nurse is the health service reconnaissance unit – an extension of the eyes and ears of the GP. Smooth communication with her is essential and her role is a very important one.

As I started home the setting sun behind me was resting on the western peaks, its slanting rays bathing the rocky summits down the Glen in golden light. Their lower slopes which swept down to the river in great curves were in shadow. Macpherson's bicycle a few miles down the road was resting against the wall, and he was casting his line along the banks of a wide pool over the places where at sundown big trout come to feed. The rocky mound between the wall and the river was once an Iron Age fort,* maybe manned anxiously by the warriors of the Glen as the news spread of the march of the Roman legions northwards up Scotland's eastern sea-board. But the legions didn't venture into the glens; to them in their camps on the plains the blue hills on their left flank must have seemed a mysterious, menacing unknown.

By now I had forgotten all about the cricket match. The hills do have this effect; their unchanging presence gives a sense of permanence which somehow dwarfs our transient hitherings and ditherings. Semi-darkness had come to the park by the time I got home; the pavilion was deserted and stumps had long since been drawn. But it might just have been a broken jaw!

---

* Archaeologists now believe that those mounds were not Iron Age forts but walled enclosures of a later date used for the cattle which came down Glenlyon on their way south from the pastures and hills of northwest Scotland.

3 Childbirth

Childbirth in an isolated practice, like other serious emergencies, often played havoc with any attempt at regular routine. When a mother for whom one had provided antenatal care went into labour, most of the other calls on one's time had to take lower precedence until the baby was safely delivered; sometimes our holidays were planned so that we would not be away at the expected time of delivery of one of our patients. The small cottage hospital obstetric unit, closed down by the Tayside Health Board in 1974, enabled us to give supervision during labour which, in such a scattered practice, would not be possible for a home delivery. A few mothers preferred to have their babies at home; most came to the cottage hospital. When the National Health Service was established in 1948, Aberfeldy hospital was designated the obstetric unit for North Perthshire. This was probably because of Jack Swanson's skill in, and enthusiasm for, obstetrics. He was already using the cottage hospital with its operating theatre for routine deliveries, and in 1962 a small extension incorporating a labour room was built.

Mothers from neighbouring practices would come to Aberfeldy to have their babies; during the 1950s about 120 deliveries per annum were carried out in the cottage hospital. This load might at times have been intolerable but for the character and ability of the late Jessie Cameron, the cottage hospital Matron. She dwelt in a flat in the hospital and lived for her work. Her capabilities as a midwife were matched by a delightful sense of humour and a capacity to make her patients and their relations feel that they were personal friends. Her skill in conducting normal labour was outstanding. She usually preferred to do the job herself without the doctor getting in the way! This saved the partnership many hours of sleep.

As a GP obstetrician Jack Swanson's touch was sure, his experience vast, and his methods sometimes 'heroic'. His policy was to shorten the second stage of labour whenever possible by forceps delivery; this was done under open-mask chloroform general anaesthesia. He would induce anaesthesia, then turn the patient on the left lateral position and hand the mask to Miss Cameron who had become a competent anaesthetist. Sitting on the delivery bed, he would check that full rotation of the baby's head had occurred, apply Milne Murray's forceps, draw the baby's head to crowning, then remove the blades and deliver manually over the perineum without doing an episiotomy.

When I first witnessed this procedure, fresh as I was from the paediatric unit of the Western General Hospital in Edinburgh, I was appalled. The use of chloroform was by then universally condemned in the academic world. But, to my surprise, the babies born under chloroform at Aberfeldy were livelier and far easier to resuscitate after delivery than those born under general anaesthesia given by a full-time anaesthetist in the Edinburgh unit. (In those days, before epidural block, inhalation anaesthesia was still the accepted routine.) Whenever possible, I acted as anaesthetist for Jack's deliveries, and concluded that, in rural practice, if general anaesthesia was to be used in childbirth, chloroform was the best agent for the job. In the late 1950s the use of pudendal block local anaesthesia, by a technique which was not difficult to master, made chloroform unnecessary for most cases of assisted delivery. It also allowed the mother to remain conscious during the birth of her baby.

Natural childbirth

In 1947 I had heard Dr Grantly Dick-Read lecture at a meeting in Edinburgh University on 'natural childbirth' and had read his book[1] on the subject with great interest. The adverse effects on normal labour of fear and tension and the method of countering these by a scheme of muscle-relaxing exercises appealed to my attitude to childbirth. Normal childbirth, without instruments and anaesthetics, was surely preferable to forceps delivery; so I offered Dick-Read relaxation exercises to mothers who came to me for antenatal care and who were interested in the method. In some cases it was brilliantly successful, but not in all; some were total failures. The reasons for failure will be discussed later in this chapter.

Mothers in Aberfeldy had come to expect a high rate of instrumental delivery under chloroform and many seemed to prefer this method. On one occasion when, in Jack Swanson's absence, I was called to one

---

1. Grantly Dick-Read, *The Revelation of Childbirth* (London, Heinemann, 1942)

of his patients in labour, she was obviously dismayed when I came into the bedroom. (She was having her second baby at home.) I dare say that word had got round that I was inclined to encourage childbirth without forceps assistance. Although in the grip of the strong contractions of second-stage labour she was making no attempt to help by bearing down; instead, as sometimes happens when mothers are overcome by fear, she was struggling and heaving, and on my arrival shouted, 'Oh! I wanted Dr Swanson with the irons and chloroform!' When I examined her, it seemed that labour was progressing perfectly normally; but she continued to shout. Somewhat exasperated, I said, 'Oh, for goodness sake, try and push.' The abruptness of my tone seemed so to surprise her that she held her breath for a moment; that did the trick by giving a little extra propulsion, the baby's head immediately appeared and the birth proceeded without any difficulty.

Technical obstetrics

During the last post-graduate teaching course which I attended at a hospital in southern England, I could not help wondering if the teaching staff did not share this mother's ignorance of such a thing as normal labour. Frequent and, to me, unnecessary inductions of labour and the wiring of women in labour to a battery of flickering dials seemed to do more harm than good.

That was in 1970; the climate of opinion about normal labour may now have changed. A movement against over-rigid regimes in hospital obstetric units, where the emotional needs of the mother in childbirth were being neglected, led in 1957 to the foundation in London of the Natural Childbirth Association. Membership of the Association increased far and wide in Britain, and, having greatly expanded its educational activities to include breast feeding and various methods of training for childbirth, in 1961 the Association achieved charitable status and was renamed the National Childbirth Trust. In many places a good relationship has been established between obstetricians and the Trust.

Food and posture

There are two crucial aspects of normal pregnancy and of natural childbirth which must never be forgotten. The first concerns food; unless a mother has been reared from her own intra-uterine days on a plentiful supply of natural food she will find it more difficult to

33

achieve a natural, unassisted labour and delivery. By 'natural food' I mean food which is varied and fresh and which has not been robbed by refining and processing of minerals, vitamins, fibre and other fresh food factors of which as yet we may be ignorant. Much of this book will be devoted to an attempt to explain to the reader what exactly is meant by 'natural food' or 'sound nutrition' and in Appendixes I and II I shall suggest practical measures for dietary change to be taken by consumers and by government.

A striking confirmation of the importance of sound nutrition in preparing the way for normal pregnancy and birth is the contrast in incidence of all the major complications of childbirth between the highest and the lowest social classes. I am sure that this sad contrast owes very little to differences in levels of medical care, but has everything to do with differences in diet.

Two nations

Women in social class five tend to be significantly smaller than those from social class one. Professor James Walker of Dundee has surveyed the stature of Scotland's women and related their performance to their height.[2] The women of the Eastern District of Glasgow are smallest of all and the evidence favours subnutrition rather than genetic factors as the cause of their small stature. The inadequately structured pelvic bones of the smaller mothers are part of the penalty of a lifetime of malnutrition. Relaxation exercises, removal of stress and sympathetic attention to a mother's emotions in labour will be of no avail in achieving a normal delivery if her pelvic bones are not adequate to allow the passage of the baby's head and shoulders.

Undernourished women have a far higher experience of congenital birth defects, prematurity and toxaemia than their well-nourished sisters in social class one. Inadequate feeding at the time of conception appears to be the main cause of these disasters.[3] The contrast in the experience of birth defect in Scotland between social class one and social class five is illustrated at fig. 2.

Magnesium and vitamin deficiencies

Toxaemia of pregnancy is associated with high blood pressure in the

---

2. J. Walker, 'Is Small Beautiful?', Scottish Office, Home and Health Department, *Health Bulletin*, vol. 36, pp. 154–61 (1978)
3. M. Wynn and A. Wynn, *Prevention of Handicap and the Health of Women* (London, Routledge and Kegan Paul, 1979), pp. 32–3

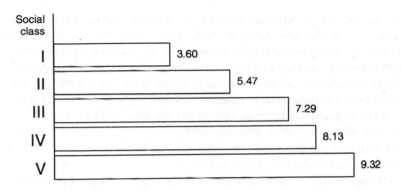

Fig. 2: *All types of malformation by social class: Scotland 1975, stillbirths plus infant deaths in first year per 1,000 live and stillbirths. Data from Registrar General for Scotland.*
(*Source:* The prevention of handicap of early pregnancy origin, *Margaret and Arthur Wynn, Foundation for Education and Research in Childbearing, London 1981*)

mother and low birth weight in the baby. Both conditions contribute to increased infant mortality which, like congenital defect, is so much more frequently encountered in social class five. Increasingly the evidence suggests dietary causes; these have been elaborated by Arthur and Margaret Wynn in a recent publication of data[4] in support of their argument that modern processed foods can be grossly deficient in magnesium and the group of B vitamins. They plead for a major trial of magnesium and vitamin supplements during pregnancy and for the addition to white flour of the magnesium removed by refining. Fig. 5 (page 59) illustrates the tremendous loss of magnesium which occurs in modern milling; a simpler measure than supplementing white flour would surely be to eat bread that had not been robbed of its magnesium in this way.

Dental decay, bone development and childbirth

The American dentist, Weston Price, in a worldwide survey[5] of dental decay during the 1930s, noted the disastrous effects of modern foods not only on the incidence of dental decay, but also on facial bone structure. Children brought up on imported, processed food, rather than on a plentiful supply of the fresh produce from their own land

4. A. Wynn and M. Wynn, 'Magnesium and other nutrient deficiencies as possible causes of hypertension and low birth weight', *Nutrition and Health*, vol. 6, no. 2 (1988), pp. 69–88
5. W. A. Price, *Nutrition and Physical Degeneration* (Los Angeles, published by author, 1939)

or sea, tended to have underdeveloped cheek bones and narrowed jawbones which caused overcrowding and overlapping of teeth. His book gives many photographs illustrating the contrast in facial appearance between children reared on traditional food and those reared on modern processed foods. One such illustration from Scotland shows the difference in appearance between family groups from the port of Stornoway on the island of Lewis, where imported processed foods were readily available, and families in the more remote island of Harris where crofters still fed their children on their own oatmeal, potatoes, fish and other local products.

It happened that shortly after reading Weston Price, I encountered a young twenty-year-old mother whose home had been on the island of Harris; she had come to live in Aberfeldy and was now pregnant for the first time. Her teeth were evenly spaced and caries free. She had broad cheek-bones and a fine general physique. Although I had never been taught that in assessing pelvic capacity in pregnancy, it would be advisable to study the patient's dental and jawbone development, I felt, in this case, that if the mother's pelvic archway was as well developed as her dental arches (and examination confirmed this indeed was so) she would have little trouble during labour.

But in the last six weeks of her pregnancy the baby turned repeatedly to a breech presentation and, in spite of attempts by the consultant, to whom the problem had been referred, to turn it back round from outside, the breech presentation remained. As a first pregnancy breech this was clearly a case for delivery in the main hospital obstetric unit, but at that time the shortage of obstetric beds in Perth Maternity Unit was acute. The mother was in any case most reluctant to go to Perth for her delivery, so with the audacity which is apt to go with youth I suggested delivery at the cottage hospital. The consultant agreed, rather reluctantly. In the event the breech delivery went with supreme ease, so my faith in inspection of the mouth and face as a means of assessing capacity for normal labour was in this case justified.

Natural positions

The second aspect of the quest for normal (or natural) childbirth which I wish to discuss, is the position of the mother during delivery. But here I must digress in an attempt to explain my use of the word 'natural'. It is a word much disliked by medical scientists because the definition of its meaning is so imprecise. Those who object to 'natural' can point out that as soon as the Neolithic people discovered how to make primitive axes with which trees could be felled, or fire which could burn forests and cook food, none of mankind's manipulation of the environment could be termed natural. And is not civilisation founded on our ability to tame and to conquer the natural world around us? Am I arguing that such blessings as anaesthesia, analgesics and assisted delivery should be withheld from women in labour? Certainly not; the advances in medical science in the last 150 years have been near miraculous. They have brought immense benefits to suffering humanity. To deny the wise use of the latest techniques of surgical or medical skill to women in labour, or to any other kind of patient, leads to the absurdities of 'Christian' Science.

But too often we forget that, in spite of all the impressive advance of medical research, the area of our ignorance is still far, far wider than that of our knowledge. The use of the word 'natural' implies a respect for the laws of nature and the need to try and understand them and to obey them.

If we look honestly at childbirth as it is conducted in probably most of our big hospitals, we would have to admit that a significant frac- tion of the difficulties which arise are due to human interference with nature's processes. Malnutrition, I repeat, in the widest sense of that term, is the most important form of interference; but I wonder if the custom of having the mother lying on her back during labour is not also an important neglect of nature's wishes.

In a review of this subject[6] published in *The Lancet* (April 1976) Dr Peter M. Dunn wrote, 'In the wake of civilisation, labour has always appeared to become more difficult, more protracted, and more painful, and I believe the main explanation may be in the posture adopted by the mother during labour'. In the course of a study of the anthropology of labour, Dr Dunn found that among some peoples, who had as yet not been influenced by 'civilised' obstetric practice (for instance the Iroquois Indians), labouring mothers squat or kneel and would vary their position according to the stage of labour.

My generation of students certainly accepted without question that labour was conducted with the mother lying on her back, supported by pillows. In this position the baby's head gets no help from gravity as it descends the birth canal; the latter tends to become slightly more narrowed than in the upright position and tears are more likely; increased pressure from the womb on the large veins leading to the

---

6. P. M. Dunn, 'Obstetric Delivery Today', *The Lancet*, 8723, vol. 1 (1990), pp. 790–3

heart may add to the risk of postpartum haemorrhage; and the uterine contractions are less efficient than in the upright position.

The reaction among obstetricians to Dr Dunn's interesting observation, if the Letters pages of *The Lancet* are a true reflection of professional opinion, was one of anger and hostility; it does seem to be difficult for some senior medical scientists to face even the remote possibility that certain techniques which they have so painfully mastered may not always be beneficial. This may also be true for those hospital staffs who rigidly adhere to long-established delivery room routines (perhaps they have changed since I retired), in which a newly born baby was given to the mother to hold for a few minutes and then whisked away to the nursery: there, after time-honoured washing, weighing and measuring, if the infant protested too much and appeared to be hungry, a glucose water feed might be given. Some people hold that this practice of giving glucose water to newly born infants sets them off on a trail of addiction to sweetened drinks.

A recent study in Sweden[7] found that successful breast-feeding was far more easily established when babies were left, immediately after birth, lying undisturbed on their mother's abdomen for at least an hour; given time and encouragement, human infants, like the young of all mammals, will find their way to the maternal nipple and start sucking. It would surely be wise in normal deliveries to give this natural process precedence over washing and weighing routines.

According to the Swedish study, early breast-feeding was less easily established in babies whose mothers had been sedated during the later stages of labour with the popular analgesic drug, pethidine; such infants, having received the drug via the placenta, were too dopey to go looking for a nipple. The authors of the study wrote:

> The conclusions to be drawn from our study are clear. First, the naked infant should be left undisturbed on the mother's abdomen until the first breast-feeding is accomplished, and the infant's efforts to take the breast actively should be promoted. Secondly, use of drugs given to the mother during labour should be restricted.[8]

All of which increases the burden of responsibility placed on doctors and nurses who have labouring mothers in their charge.

---

7. R. Lennart and M. O. Alade, 'Effect of delivery room routines on success of first breast feed', *The Lancet*, vol. 336 (1990), pp. 1105–1107
8. *Ibid.*, p. 1107

4 Convertible Births

After learning about the disadvantages of birth with the mother lying on a labour bed, I often regretted that our cottage hospital obstetric unit was closed before Aberfeldy mothers could have the chance of trying alternative methods, particularly those of the well-known French doctor, Michel Odent. I had the privilege of meeting Dr Odent at a conference in 1978. He uses labour rooms so designed and furnished that the mother, in the later stages of labour, can position herself as she pleases; usually her baby is born with her standing, supported by helpers or husband. Dr Odent is convinced that this method ensures easier deliveries and a much reduced risk of lacerations during the birth of the baby's head. I cannot, however, find much enthusiasm for his other method, whereby delivery occurs with mother sitting or kneeling in a warm bath, so that the infant emerges under water – surely a somewhat unusual way for us to enter this world!

The following diary entry tells how my only experience of conducting labour with the mother sitting upright, as on a chair, was quite unplanned:

Spring 1958. There seemed to be no particular urgency about the call this morning, to see Mrs Wright. The visiting list was surprisingly short, so I hoped for time to browse through unopened copies of the *British Medical Journal*. Mrs Wright lived down the river; as she was due for delivery at the end of her second pregnancy in about three weeks I decided to go early.

It was a lovely morning as I set out without a care in the world. Sun sparkled on the winding river; green leaf was everywhere breaking the bonds of a cold spring and the salmon fishers in the blue-painted boat made a pretty picture as they trawled up and down the big corner pool. My carefree thoughts of spring abruptly vanished when, on crossing the threshold, I heard the unmistakable expulsive gasp of a mother in labour.

Mrs Wright was booked for delivery at the cottage hospital; examination confirmed that she was indeed near the second stage of labour; either we should carry on here or make a dash for the hospital. The road by the river winds and twists but the distance was only about four and a half miles; we should make the hospital in ten minutes; so with the help of the district nurse, Mrs Wright was quickly made as comfortable as possible in the front passenger seat of my car, a Morris Minor convertible. The road, I repeat, twists; at every corner her contractions seemed to get stronger. But at last we rounded the final bend and were in sight of the town and the haven of the little hospital on the hill. Just as I was about to give a sigh of relief, she said, 'Doctor, I think it's coming'.

I drew into a driveway entrance; the baby's head was indeed near point of delivery and there was nothing for it but to proceed with the birth. I took off my jacket, rolled up my sleeves and, standing on the road, leaned across the driver's seat to control the birth of the head; the steering wheel tended to get in the way, otherwise the method presented no difficulty. Mrs Wright was a model patient; she sat outwardly quite unperturbed and pushed or rested when I asked her to do so. The birth was supremely easy; the silly words of a silly song came unbidden to my mind, 'Why don't we do this more often'.

The baby, although small, was vigorous and of a good colour; the placenta could wait, so giving the lustily crying baby to her mother to hold, I started up and continued the journey. 'Are you all right?' I asked, glancing at my passenger. The fright from what I saw came near to making me lose control and plunge into the ditch.

Mrs Wright, still composed and uncomplaining, held the baby on her lap; above the baby was the unmistakable curve of a still occupied womb. Steering with my right hand, I used my left to carry out a hasty palpation, which confirmed that we had indeed another unsuspected passenger. As if to put the matter beyond doubt, Mrs Wright announced that again she wanted to push.

By this time were approaching Wade's bridge; as my little car threaded its way through the main street, I tried to nod and smile to familiar faces as if nothing unusual was happening. The car hood was, mercifully, up, so spectators could not see what was happening nor hear my anguished plea to my patient, 'Please try not to push!' At the hospital I seized one of the wheeled chairs usually parked by the porch and with the help of an astonished nurse, got both mother and baby to the labour ward; the breech of the second twin was already appearing; the birth was as easy and troublefree as the first. The twins throve normally and Mrs Wright seemed none the worse for her ordeal.

On ruefully reviewing this case at the time I was somewhat comforted to know that in days before routine ultrasound scanning, even consultants might occasionally miss the diagnosis of a twin pregnancy. It is easy to be wise after the event and wrong to blame circumstances for one's failings, but in a scattered practice, where the mother has not access to public or private transport, arrangements for regular antenatal examinations, which are so essential in obstetric care, sometimes broke down. In this case, for want of transport, two of the early appointments had been missed; I had indeed noted in the antenatal record card the possibility of a twin pregnancy, but this had not been pursued.

It was with considerable envy that I observed, when attending refresher courses at large maternity hospitals, how, at the request of the antenatal staff, an ambulance would bring a mother for her appointment and take her home. The regulations of the NHS forbade a GP to use an ambulance to bring a patient to his consulting rooms even for antenatal examinations. I like to think that had such a transport system been available, the twins would not have been missed.

The decision to make for the hospital turned out to be wrong. We should have stayed quietly at home; the longer my experience of obstetrics, the less able I felt accurately to forecast the time of delivery! If the doctor did not come out of this episode with much credit, there is no doubt that the heroine was Mrs Wright, who remained so calm during what for her must have been a very trying car journey.

The easy delivery in the sitting position may have been due to the small size of the twin (about 6 lbs); but in the hope of trying out this method for scientific assessment, I wondered if there might be a case for fitting Morris Minor front seats in the labour rooms of some of our teaching hospitals!

41

5 Work, Leisure and Fatigue

In drafting a new partnership agreement in 1948, my request for a regular half-day off in the week was, I felt, seen by my senior partner as a sign of the decadence of the new breed of general practitioners. Systems of time off did not appeal to his generation and would have been impossible to fit into a medical-political programme. In many practices of the pre-war era, the absence of any arrangement for ensuring regular opportunities for leisure was dictated by economic forces; practices were often small and single-handed; incomes were mostly low, so it was essential, especially when a community was served by two rival practices, as was the case for a while in Aberfeldy, to be permanently available in case a patient might be lost to a rival. Better security of income under the NHS was to change this attitude.

In Aberfeldy there had been talk of reviving the Breadalbane Cricket Club; it had lapsed during the war, and during my first summer I had joined a few cricket enthusiasts in making plans to raise cash and to lay a new square in Victoria Park. In the hope of playing regularly, Saturday was my choice of half-day. My partner, Jack, readily agreed to this but the system was bound to be difficult because, as has already been explained, Saturday tended to be a hectic day. On many occasions, especially before we engaged an assistant, I had to leave the field in order to attend emergencies in hospital or elsewhere.

Hydroelectric schemes

From 1952 to 1958 important developments in the field of hydroelectricity greatly added to the clinical responsibilities of the practice. A series of dams and generation stations were built in Glen Lyon and Lochtayside; wooden hutted camps housing some 700–800 workers were constructed at Cashlie, Stronuich and Lubreoch, all at the west end of Glen Lyon, and almost thirty miles from Aberfeldy. More permanent houses were built or found for managers and engineers and their families. The firms involved were helpful in providing transport for sick or injured employees, but inevitably this intrusion greatly added to our problems in providing a twenty-four-hour service.

Our practice, without the hydroelectric employees, totalled around 3,600 and, as described in an earlier chapter, the cottage hospital received obstetric cases from surrounding practices. As the following diary entries suggest, to be on duty single-handed for this load even for a day was at times daunting.

August 1957, Monday. Jack away on holiday. The phone never stops ringing; saw thirty-five patients at consulting today, which is a lot for this practice; feel bleary-eyed with fatigue. There have been emergencies almost daily in the last ten days to distant places. The worst of it is the crushing feeling of suffocation by work and a kind of mental strangulation which leaves you no time to think.

Tuesday. We reached a kind of climax today, starting at 7.15 a.m. with a summons to the hospital for a Mrs Smith, in labour, who was failing to complete her second stage. A patient of Dr X whom I had not seen before; was annoyed that I had not been called sooner, as she had been too long in second stage. As I arrived at the hospital a stretcher, bearing a workman with a very badly broken leg, was brought in from the hydro-scheme. Called the assistant to help, did a low forceps delivery under pudendal block anaesthesia. Placenta then retained, so had to give chloroform and do manual removal, after which there was a brisk postpartum haemorrhage. Put up a drip and sent to Perth for blood. At this point Sister came hurrying with a message that Dr Douglas Mackay had had a heart attack and requested urgently to be visited at home. Mrs Smith stable; stopped bleeding and seems in good shape. Plasma drip going well, and blood should arrive soon. Baby also mercifully vigorous and in good shape. Visited Dr Mackay; he is getting very frail but no signs of infarction; said I would look back as soon as possible. Got home about 9.30 to shave and have breakfast and learnt that a visit was required to Stronuich camp (nearly thirty miles away). The visiting list was terribly long already; had hardly finished breakfast when Mrs Inglis of Craigend Cottage at Glen Lyon phoned to say that her youngest (age two) had got hold of an unidentified bottle in the shed, had drunk from it and was now screaming and vomiting. A few minutes later a message came in from the local circus to say that the manager of the circus had collapsed and wanted a doctor urgently.

My memory of these days is of a constant struggle against fatigue. A curious aspect of such fatigue is its addictive effect. Other GPs with whom I have discussed this agree that it does occur. The overworked doctor (and I am sure this applies to other trades and professions) finds it somehow easier to go on working than to stop and do something else. I noticed frequently in the 1950s that when my half-day came along, in a strange way I almost wished more calls would come in, so that I would have to go on working. This habit probably begins when the pressure of work, bit by bit, leads to the shedding of non-professional interests, hobbies and other activities. Another factor which makes it difficult for some GPs to stop working is the seductive effect of having one's ego repeatedly boosted by being wanted; this leads to a reluctance to be unavailable or to let a colleague take over. 'Workaholic', when applied to General Practitioners therefore, may have some scientific basis.

During the war, a combination of sleep deprivation, mental and muscular fatigue, fear and the horror of what was happening, often made strong men weep like children. I remember vividly a battalion company commander taking me aside on one terrible day of battle to ask me how he could stop himself bursting into tears in front of his men. This request surprised me, as he had always seemed to be a hard disciplinarian, lacking in sensitivity. But it was no place for prolonged discussion on the subject. My only comfort was to tell him that that was exactly how I felt myself, which was true; this brief revelation of mutual anguish was maybe of some comfort to both of us, since we were able to resume our various duties.

It would be wrong to give the impression that during the 1950s spare time was non-existent. Slack days did occur. I was usually able to enjoy my Saturday cricket in summer, and in winter Sonia and I found the snow of Ben Lawers gave a wonderful escape from daily toil. As winter snows filled the high gullies, whenever possible, usually on a Sunday, we would pack our rucksacks with the ingredients of lunch and, often with friends from Aberfeldy, make for the Loch-na-Larig road, which winds up the side of the Edramucky burn to a level of about 1500 feet before it dips down to Glen Lyon. When the snow cover allowed, we could drive up the road to its highest point (in the early years there was no proper car park), don our skis and climb, using skins on the undersurface of the skis, to the Scottish Ski Club hut on Ben Ghlas. In those days the hut was a regular meeting place for the Scottish Ski Club, and attempts at primitive tows with temperamental engines were made by a heroic group of enthusiasts. But mostly we had to climb on our two legs in order to enjoy the downhill runs. In Scotland winter snows seldom fall, as in the Alps, vertically. Blizzards usually come with strong winds which pile the snow into the gullies made by the burns, and often blow it off the ridges. Ski runs therefore are comparatively narrow and often separated by heather, peat or rock.

The following little poem appeared in the Scottish Club Journal some time in the 1950s:

> We ski in every kind of weather,
> On wet snow, dry snow, rocks and heather,
> But when we ski in muddy pools
> We're bluddy fools.

Occasionally if there had been a really deep fall of snow and the hill roads were blocked, skis were a help in visiting distant cottages, as I shall describe later on.

'Of the earth, earthy'

Fatigue from the pressure of medical work in the 1950s was, from time to time, made somewhat worse by struggles to grow as much as possible of our own family food, using organic or biological methods. This stemmed from a conviction that unwise use of the land was one of the factors leading to the declining health and vitality of the Scottish people. Research by a distinguished botanist, Sir Albert Howard,[1] suggested a unity in the health of the soil, the health of plants, and the health of humanity; soil fertility was dependent on biological forces, so the life in the soil could not be separated from the life of men. I had also been deeply impressed by Lady Eve Balfour's book *The Living Soil*,[2] which introduced me to the work of Sir Robert McCarrison[3] and opened up a field of knowledge and a view of health and disease never dreamt of in my medical studies at university. All over the strath of the upper Tay and in Glen Lyon silent ruins reminded us of the time when most of the food for the people living there came from their own land. Now the bulk of food was imported; the variety

---

1. A. Howard, *Farming and Gardening in Health and Disease* (London, Faber, 1945)
2. E. B. Balfour, *The Living Soil* (London, Faber, 1943)
3 R. McCarrison, *Nutrition and Health* (London, Faber, 1961)

and quality of vegetables in the 1950s was poor.* Many of my patients seemed to live by opening cans. So my wife and I set out to remedy the dearth of fresh vegetables by growing our own.

The garden plot

I knew little of horticulture, but determined to master the art of compost making in the hope that the rest would follow. At this time (1950) wartime rationing had not yet ended, so we established a hen run at the bottom of the garden and dug a vegetable plot out of part of the lawn. A trailer behind the Austin Ten car enabled me to collect grass cuttings from the putting green down the road – no selective hormone weedkillers in those days. Bracken, nettles or the odd load of cow dung were easily obtained; the composts made from these materials along with hen dung soon gave impressive results. But I was occasionally reminded that if you spend all your day sitting in your car or at a desk, and then go forking binfuls of heavy compost, your back is apt to protest or seize up altogether! Gardening can be relaxing and refreshing, but when, repeatedly, you are called away from the vegetable plot to cope with some emergency, the result tends to frustration and fatigue. We began experimenting with Chase cloches and discovered that autumn-sown lettuces, even here in the Highlands, could be ready for cutting by the end of April.

Delusions of grandeur

The success of the garden plot gave rise to a rather daft dream to do the thing on a larger scale, not for any commercial profit, but to demonstrate that health-giving food could come from local soil and could be grown without the use of soluble chemicals or toxic sprays. The garden behind our house, Inzievar, at the crossroads, got little sun in the early part of the year; across the river in the south-facing slopes the mean temperature was higher than in the town, where winter frosts lingered. The owner of a small sheltered field which had once been part of one of the Boltachan crofts gave me permission to cultivate it. My accountant with whom I had discussed the 'market garden' idea explained that the tax laws then prevailing allowed hobby gardeners or hobby farmers to offset losses against income tax; provided I made a big enough loss in the first year, I would not be worse off. So we cast around for a gardener; a full-time employee was

---

* In recent years, the variety and quality of fresh fruit and vegetables in our shops has greatly improved; but they are very expensive in the Highlands.

essential. In March 1959 I came across James, a sixteen-year-old school leaver, whose family had recently come to Aberfeldy. He was a cheerful chap and seemed keen to be enrolled as a chauffeur-gardener at £5 weekly.

We invested in a pack of Chase's commercial barn cloches, and a Landmaster rotovator; the field was fenced and from the saw-mill's cast-off timber James built a hen house to take forty point-of-lay pullets and a large compost bin. By autumn, we were ready to make our first sowing of lettuces and sweet peas – a row of peas between two rows of lettuces to fit the width of a cloche. The lettuces always seemed to grow better when 'companioned' with sweet peas.

Lettuces, peas, beans, strawberries, carrots, sweet peas and various other crops in time did well, and there was no difficulty in finding buyers for the produce and for the eggs; but the demands of general practice and the crises of gardening on this scale led to crazy situations, as my diary relates:

Winter 1960. It was rather a long labour; I felt I could not depart from the hospital labour room until the baby had arrived. A tremendous gale was blowing when I emerged from the hospital at about 2 a.m. As often happens when overtired and keyed up after the anxiety of birth, my mind was overactive and sleep would not come. I had returned to bed and was listening to sheets of rain smashing against the west-facing window when, with dismay, I remembered we had not yet secured a long row of cloches. The whole lot were in danger of destruction in a gale such as this; they would have to be secured. Sonia felt I had taken leave of my senses when I rose from bed and said I must go across to the garden.

Perhaps in moments of extreme fatigue associated with lack of sleep the mind is capable of sudden clarity and of coming near to answering the prayer of Robert Burns:

> Oh! Would some power the giftie gie us
> To see ourselves as others see us.

There I was, in a state of near drunkenness with fatigue, in the pitch dark wearing Wellington boots and an overcoat over pyjamas, up to the ankles in mud; drenching rain and a fierce gale added to total misery. I realised, with awful certainty, that had any of my colleagues in psychiatry beheld this scene, they would swiftly have sent for an ambulance and two strong men in white coats!

Another incident added to suspicions that doctoring and market gardening do not easily combine: bailie Peter McGregor, proprietor of the fish, flower and vegetable shop, phoned one day to ask if my sweet peas were ready and could our garden supply him with a few bunches, which it could and did. I later learned with alarm that the flowers were required to make a wreath for a patient of mine who had died in the cottage hospital. Would the General Medical Council, I wondered, have something to say to a GP with a commercial interest in wreath-making?

After some eighteen months, James discovered that he could earn more than twice as much as we could afford to pay him by driving a lorry at a west coast hydroelectric scheme; so he was off. We continued cultivating the field with part-time labour for a couple of years, but then the tax concessions for gardening were (to the eternal shame of the government of the day) stopped. So the 'market garden' had to be abandoned, but I did not regret attempting a project which, when the motives for it are understood, was in keeping with the prime objective of the National Health Service – to prevent disease. I remain convinced that unless land use is seen as part of health promotion, not only in Scotland but throughout the world, costly medical services will not make people healthier.

African example

If I had possessed the drive and ability of Dr Halley Stott, I might have persuaded others, as he did, to join in establishing a demonstration organic garden. Dr Stott, a graduate of Edinburgh University Medical School (1935), lived at Botha's Hill at Natal in South Africa, beside a large Zulu reserve called the Valley of a Thousand Hills. He became so concerned about the level of malnutrition and disease in the families whose hutted homes and 'crofts' were scattered over this lovely tract of land, that he bought a hundred acres bordering the reserve and then left his medical practice in order to found a 'Socio-Medical Experiment'[4] for the promotion of health among his new Zulu neighbours. The backbone of the experiment is the medical service based in the Botha's Hill Health Centre, which in January 1951 was established with the cooperation of the State Health Department.

Dr Stott was convinced that the deteriorating health and social disintegration of a once proud and vigorous people were due to their inability to change from a semi-nomadic, shifting agriculture to a

4. H. H. Stott, 'The Valley Trust', *Journal of the Soil Association*, vol. 10, no. 5 (January 1959)

static life which required the disciplines of settled agriculture. 'Great dependence was placed on the trading store with its supplies of refined maize products and other processed foods such as cake flour, white bread and commercial sugar, all of little or no nutritional value. Accompanying this were bad cooking practices, serious soil neglect and misuse with a negligible local production of foods containing nutrients essential for health'.[5] A large demonstration garden was created beside the Health Centre, as was a Nutrition Education hut; both are staffed by enthusiastic Zulu demonstrators, who teach families how to grow and prepare health-giving food. Zulu health visitors, several large communal gardens and new technology for clean water and sound sanitation are features of this inspiring project, now known as the Valley Trust. Only organic methods are taught; Dr Stott has strenuously resisted attempts by some advisers to introduce chemical fertilisers. When Sonia and I visited the Valley Trust in 1985, we sensed the dedication and enthusiasm of the staff, especially the agricultural demonstrator, a staunch advocate of the use of composts for his terraced plots. The climate, people, soil and social conditions of the Perthshire Scots are quite different from those of the Natal Zulus, but the underlying problem of malnutrition is the same.

It became increasingly clear that I could not continue large-scale vegetable and fruit growing and do justice to the demands of our patients. By that time (1959) I had been in the practice for over ten years; my life was entwined with many families in the role of family doctor, a relationship I did not want to abandon. I therefore decided to limit our growing to the needs of the family.

Now that Dr Ann Thomson had joined the partnership, more consulting room space was badly needed; space was created in 1963 by turning the ground floor of Inzievar into a consulting suite, when our family, now enlarged by the arrival of two boys and a girl, moved to a new bungalow built on a hill known as the 'fort'. In case important prehistoric remains might be destroyed, the hill top had to be excavated before the bungalow could be built. But although the archaeologists found no signs of fortified dwellings, they uncovered a small part of what may once have been a prehistoric stone wall round the top of the hill and a lot of metallic chunks, remnants of an eighteenth-century bloomery, where local charcoal was used for smelting iron.

The hill is a glacial deposit of stones and boulders covered by a fairly thin soil; the vegetable-growing plots had to be levelled and

5. H. H. Stott, *Biological Priorities in Rural Health*: The Valley Trust, Botha's Hill, Natal, S. Africa (1980)

terraced; in spite of the stones and exposure to west winds, yields and quality seemed excellent, thanks, I am sure, to the generous treatment with composts.

6 Varicose Veins

Sonia and I got out of the car because it would go no further; the snow was almost a foot deep, and at this gradient even our new winter tyres were spinning and sliding.

We put on our skis and started climbing. The moor road, dug out of the side of the hill in the days when there was much traffic between the village far below us and the shielings or peat cuttings on the moor above, takes a hairpin bend here and gets much steeper. Ahead of us the snow was moulded over the line of the road in huge drifts, shaped by the wind into fantastic curves so that climbing was hard work. But with skins strapped to the undersurface of the skis a climber can often get over deep snow with ease and rapidity. Nowadays, thanks to the proliferation of ski tows and chair lifts, Scottish skiers seldom bother to ascend this hard way and how much they miss! We emerged from a line of trees on to the hill park enclosed by stone walls, and now we could hardly follow the road at all; in some places drifts covered the walls so that we could easily cross and re-cross them. Soon we were over the top wall and on to the moor; in front of us was our objective, a lesser peak of some 1800 feet, and away to our right, looking lonely and desolate, stood High Ridge Farm with its steading and sheep fank. The slopes of our peak which curved down to the hill park were covered with vast unbroken stretches of snow, piled on this, the lee side of the hill, to depths of six, eight or ten feet – firm and smooth, ideal for either ascent or descent on skis.

As we got higher the whole glen was spread before us in all its splendour. From time to time the snowstorms of January are followed by still days of sunshine and frost, and what a magic world of whiteness rewards those who, at this time of year, explore the hills. Beyond the hill, the moor stretched on a wide plateau to a rugged skyline of higher peaks and as we paused, breathless from the long climb, nothing seemed to move or live in this petrified ocean of snow. There was no wind, all was silence except for the thumping of one's heart. But as we listened a faint tinkling spoke of a burn, still running, away down under the snow. A movement ahead caught my eye and I could make out a white hare. Startled by our intrusion, he loped along for a step or two, then sat bolt upright, listening, a tiny pillar of white merging perfectly with the landscape.

Having reached our summit we took off our skis and unpacked coffee and sandwiches; lunch in these surroundings is a feast for the gods. But we couldn't linger long for, even without wind, the edge of the frost was keen and the sun would soon disappear behind the ridge on the opposite side of the glen.

Our descent was, as always, hilarious – exhilarating on the smooth firm snow near the top where turning was easy, but chaotic on the thinner crusted surface below. A final 'schuss' across the hill park took us to the High Ridge steading. This routine visit to Mrs McBeen, the wife of the shepherd, had been left for Sunday so that we could make an expedition of it. The reason for the visit was to have a look at her varicose ulcer and to change the supporting paste bandage with which it was being treated. We left our skis at the back door and went in. Mrs McBeen, a wiry active little person of about fifty-five, had a delightful conditioned reflex; whenever a visitor came into the kitchen, she would immediately hurry to the stove to put the kettle on. I suppose that at High Ridge, often isolated for weeks in winter, the arrival of a visitor was something to be celebrated. On weekdays, it sometimes seemed that no matter at what time of the day one visited High Ridge, the postman had got there first and was drinking his tea by the fire.

Fruit cake, scones and cheese were hastily produced before we could get down to the business of cutting off the old bandage and applying a new one. While this was going on, Mr McBeen sat in the corner working away with his knife, hazel stick and tup horn from which, in the dark winter evenings, he fashioned beautiful shepherds' crooks.

The deep, weeping, elongated ulcer on the inner surface of Mrs McBeen's left lower leg was now causing little discomfort and was slowly healing. Both her legs were disfigured by huge bunches of varicose veins. Supporting bandages had to be changed weekly or fortnightly over long and tedious weeks; but usually in the end this treatment did seem to promote healing. Our visiting list invariably included two or three cases like this one.

Outside, the approach of twilight, which comes so swiftly in the short January days, reminded us that it would not do to be out on the moor in darkness; so we drained our cups and skied gingerly over the deep snow to the road. The frost was as keen as ever as we reached the car.

In human suffering, disability, lost production and medical care, the cost of varicose veins must be enormous. A recent estimate of the total number of cases of the common complication of varicose veins, varicose ulcer, an example of which we had just seen, gives a figure of 150,000 in the UK, with the financial cost at £300-£600 million.[1]

The cause of varicose veins, or the possibility of prevention, was certainly never thought of in medical education. By by 1960 I was convinced that the researches of Sir Robert McCarrison gave a true explanation of the cause of many of the diseases encountered in our practice. McCarrison's research in India[2] had been inspired by his observation, as an officer of the old Colonial Medical Service, of the health, vigour and longevity of certain northern races among whom he worked. He concluded that the contrast in health between these isolated races and the diseased populations of the industrial West was due, more than any other factor, to the increasing consumption in the West of processed unnatural foods, particularly white flour and refined sugar.

It had evidently never occurred to doctors seeking prevention that varicose veins might simply be a complication of constipation and therefore linked to the consumption of refined carbohydrate foods.

Thanks to my participation in a brief discussion in the correspondence columns of the *British Medical Journal* in 1960, I was to meet T. L. Cleave whose enquiring mind cast a new light on the cause and prevention of many of the serious diseases which bring untold suffering and disability to twentieth-century Britain.

In 1960, two booklets, one on bread, the other on sugar, issued by the British Medical Association for guidance of families,[3] stated that plenty of refined sugar was good for children and that white bread was every bit as nourishing as wholemeal. I protested in a letter to the *British Medical Journal*[4] and quoted McCarrison's work in support of my argument. A few days after my letter appeared in February 1960, I received a letter, written in rather spidery hand writing, signed by T. L. Cleave, who expressed agreement with my views and informed me that he was about to publish a book showing how the

1. Unsigned article, 'High Compression Bandaging Heals Venous Ulcers', *BMJ*, vol. 297 (1988), p. 1142
2. R. McCarrison, *Nutrition and Health* (London, Faber, 1961)
3. British Medical Association Family Doctor Booklets, 1960
4. W. W. Yellowlees, ' "Family Doctor" on Food', Letter to the *BMJ*, 5170, vol. 1 (1960), pp. 426–7

consumption of fibre-depleted foods such as white flour and sugar caused varicose veins. This idea was surely absurd; T. L. C., I thought, was just another of those daft enthusiasts who become possessed of strange ideas about food and health. How could refined carbohydrates like white flour and refined sugar possibly cause varicose veins?

Soon after an initial exchange of letters, a slim booklet, 'On the cause of Varicose Veins and their Prevention and Arrest by Natural Means',[5] arrived by post, sent with the compliments of Surgeon Captain T. L. Cleave. Having a desk top permanently cluttered with unread journals, I was about to thrust aside yet more reading matter, but a glance at the opening pages compelled further attention. The simple clarity of the writing, the author's scholarship and the logic of the argument could not be ignored. Here was new evidence which fully confirmed McCarrison's research and which must be explored.

---

5. T. L. Cleave, *On the Causation of Varicose Veins* (Bristol, John Wright, 1960)
Note: In these and all succeeding notes, the abbreviation *BMJ* is used to refer to the *British Medical Journal*.

7 Surgeon-Captain T. L. Cleave

In the years that followed my introduction to Surgeon Captain T. L. Cleave, until his death in 1983, I was privileged to be among the circle of doctors, scientists and writers who enjoyed continuing friendship and correspondence with this remarkable man. He never failed to answer my queries by replying in letters expressed in eloquent and stimulating language, always written in longhand, the important parts being underlined or written in green or red ink. On several occasions I was able to continue our discussions during brief visits to the home of Helen and Peter (as he was always known, although his Christian names were Thomas Latimer) at Fareham. Helen was a kind hostess and devoted wife whose support throughout Peter's unceasing campaign was of invaluable help to him. Reared in Cornwall, he had been a precocious student, completing his studies at Bristol University Medical School between the ages of sixteen and twenty-one. He and his brother Hugh gave lifelong service as doctors in the Royal Navy.

He was first and foremost a conscientious clinician, deeply concerned with the health of his naval patients; the driving force in his work was a burning desire to understand causes and so teach prevention; this desire may well have been fired by the tragic loss of a young sister who died at an early age from acute appendicitis.

Cleave possessed intuitive skills in understanding the ways of beasts, birds and and fish. He saw that animals were perfectly adapted to their food supply as it occurred in nature, and that although they preyed on each other they did not suffer in the wild from the degenerative diseases (such as cancer), which now so plague human beings. Man, too, he was convinced, was perfectly adapted to his food supply as it occurred in nature; after long thought and study of the diet and health of populations throughout the world, he concluded that the occurrence of certain degenerative diseases was simply due to the way

55

in which human beings altered their natural food, above all by refining their carbohydrates.

He was able to put his theories to the test in his clinical work in the navy, and before retiring in 1957 he spent four years as Director of Research at the Royal Naval medical school. After retiring, he continued his nutrition research and devoted his energy to writing, in the hope of making his professional colleagues aware of the tremendous importance of his thesis. Ornithology was one of his hobbies; another was organic gardening and the growing of fruit and vegetables in his impressive garden at Fareham. The implication of carbohydrate refining still seems to be so little understood, both by consumers and by doctors, that I feel it is essential to state here in the simplest possible terms the basis of Cleave's teaching.

Sugars and starches

Carbohydrates in the form of sugars and starches provide the human race with much of its energy; these foods, created by the action of sunlight on the green pigment (chlorophyl) of plant leaves, and then stored in fruit, stem or root, are the simplest and the most direct agents by which the sun's energy is made available for the diverse needs of the human body. More complex forms of carbohydrates exist in the indigestible cellulose or lignin, and other supporting structures which help to form the plant.

As human food, starches and sugars are broken down in the stomach and small intestine and ultimately absorbed into the blood stream in the form of the simplest carbohydrate molecule – glucose. Glucose is then used in three ways by the body.[1] It is 'burned' to give energy for the work of human tissues; it is stored in the liver as glycogen; and it is stored as fat, some of which circulates in the blood.

Sugar

Fig. 3 shows a sugar-bearing plant (sugar beet, carrot, beetroot, parsnip); the small shaded area represents the store of sugar which, by industrial refining, can be separated from the parent plant.

A portion of, let us say, beetroot weighing 100 grams would yield, in this way, a small teaspoonful of sugar (10 grams). In order to eat from this natural source the few teaspoonfuls of sugar commonly added to tea or coffee, we would have to eat about a pound of beetroot, and in order to eat the sugar ration consumed daily by the average

---

1. R. McDowall, *Handbook of Physiology and Biochemistry* (London, John Murray, 1955), p. 361

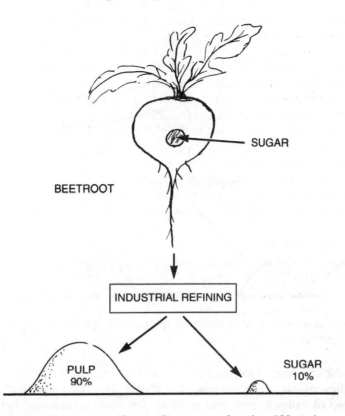

Fig. 3: *Industrial extraction of sugar from parent plant (per 100 gm.)*
(Source: author)

citizen (140 grams) we would have to consume four to six beetroot.
The check on appetite from a full stomach would make this impossible,
thus consumption of the quantities of sugar being eaten today could
not occur from natural sources; consumption of refined sugar has been
made possible only by the use, firstly of slaves, then of machines.

This is the crux of Cleave's teaching; when we eat refined sugar or
flour we are asking our bodies to cope with a substance which does
not exist in nature – a substance made available only by industrial
refining; natural sources of sugar always include, with the plant tissues, vitamins, minerals, fibre, protein and various other substances;
honey, as we shall see, is the nearest natural equivalent to refined
sugar but it, too, contains traces of vitamins, minerals, wax and protein. Refined sugar separated from its parent plant is thus rightly said

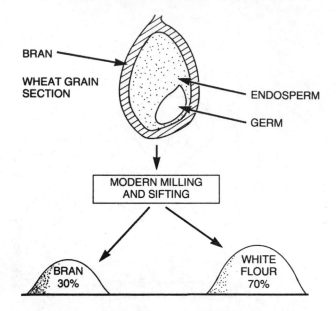

BRAN

WHEAT GRAIN
SECTION

ENDOSPERM

GERM

MODERN MILLING
AND SIFTING

BRAN
30%

WHITE
FLOUR
70%

Fig. 4: *Alteration of wheat by milling to produce 70% extraction flour (Source: author)*

to consist of 'empty calories' and so children who consume enormous quantities of sugar as sweets, ice cream and in other forms are deprived of valuable nutrients required for normal health and growth.

Starch
Fig. 4 illustrates the refining process applied to wheat grains. Separation of starch from the parent plant is not as total as in the case of refined sugar; refined flour does contain reduced amounts of essential nutrients, but it is an impoverished food; fig. 5, based on data from the book entitled *Bread*,[2] illustrates the enormous loss of minerals and vitamins when wheat flour is refined.

Until recent decades, the few doctors who deplored the degrading of wheat flour in this way were ignored or derided; the loss of vital nutrients through the industrial refining of sugar cane (or beet) and of wheat grains during the last two hundred years has had a dire effect on the stature and general health especially of poorer sections of the population, who depend on white flour for most of their calories.[3]

2. Lord Horder, C. Dodds and T. Moran, *Bread* (London, Constable, 1954)
3. J. C. Drummond and A. Wilbraham, *The Englishman's Food* (Alden Press, 1939), chap. XXII

Surgeon-Captain T. L. Cleave

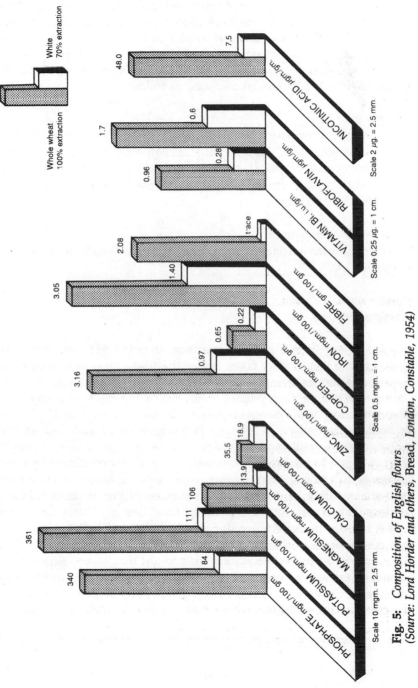

Fig. 5: *Composition of English flours*
(Source: Lord Horder and others, Bread, London, Constable, 1954)

It is easy to understand the harmful effects of refining through loss of essential vitamins and minerals; but Cleave's unique contribution to our knowledge of the cause of modern diseases lay in his demonstration of three mechanisms at work which have nothing to do with vitamin or mineral deficiency; each of the three mechanisms results in three separated groups of diseases, as follows:[4]

By removal of fibre
   a. Simple constipation with its complications of venous ailments (varicose veins, deep venous thrombosis, haemorrhoids and varicocele); diverticular disease and, in part, cancer of the colon.
   b. Dental caries (in conjunction with the taking of sugar) and peridontal disease.

From overconsumption
Diabetes, obesity, coronary thrombosis, primary E coli infections and gallstones.

From removal of protein
Peptic ulceration.

It will be seen from the above headings that the varicose veins discussed in the last chapter come under the first group of diseases due to constipation caused by removal of fibre. Cleave was the first doctor to advocate the obvious treatment of the near universal state of constipation of the bowels of industrial societies; his naval patients on board ship had no access to wholewheat bread and had limited rations of fresh fruits and vegetables, so he brought aboard a supply of wheat bran, to be taken for the relief and prevention of constipation. Unprocessed wheat bran simply replaces roughage, removed by industrial refining, and such was the success of this treatment during the last war on board the battleship *King George V* that there was unrest among the crew when the supply of bran failed!

A tablespoonful of unprocessed bran taken once or twice daily in milk, soup or with any other food, as advised by Cleave, transformed the lives of many of my patients plagued by constipation. My wife and I never depart on a holiday, during which we will be at the mercy of refined carbohydrates, without taking a good supply of bran.

---

4. T. L. Cleave, *The Saccharine Disease* (Bristol, John Wright, 1974)

The saccharine disease

The diseases listed above in three groups, although very different in their manifestation, all have one simple cause – the refining of carbohydrate-bearing crops. In their diversity they can be compared with a disease like tuberculosis which has one simple cause – infection by the tubercule bacillus – but many different manifestations in the human body.

Cleave suggested that his three groups of diseases would best be seen as different manifestations of one master disease if the latter was named 'the saccharine disease', that is, a disease related to sugary sweetness. Fig. 6 illustrates how widely in the human body are spread the manifestations of this disease.

In the 1950s and 60s Cleave expressed his views forcibly and lucidly in many letters and articles in the medical press, but these made very little impact and often his theories were ridiculed. In 1966 together with G. D. Campbell he published his first comprehensive textbook, *Diabetes, Coronary Thrombosis and the Saccharine Disease.*[5] In a foreword to this book, Sir Richard Doll, Director of the Statistical Research Unit of the Medical Research Council and Regius Professor of Medicine at Oxford, wrote 'whether the predictions that Surgeon-Captain Cleave and Dr Campbell make in this book will prove to be correct remains to be seen but if only a small part of them do, the authors will have made a bigger contribution to medicine than most university departments or medical research units make in the course of a generation'.

In 1969, a third author, Dr N. S. Painter, joined Cleave and Campbell in the publication of a second edition; Dr Painter contributed a separate chapter on diverticular disease.

Cleave and Burkitt

Peter Cleave did not relish making speeches; he preferred evenings by the river with sea trout rod to the camaraderie of medical meetings. He communicated better by the written than by the spoken word and did not easily make human relationships. He tended to be outspoken in his criticisms of those who disagreed with him; years of ridicule and neglect may well have soured his approach to professional colleagues.

However, in 1967 a new voice was heard in the debate on the cause of degenerative or non-infective diseases. In that year the late Mr

5. T. L. Cleave, G. D. Campbell, *Diabetes, Coronary Thrombosis and the Saccharine Disease* (Bristol, John Wright, 1966)

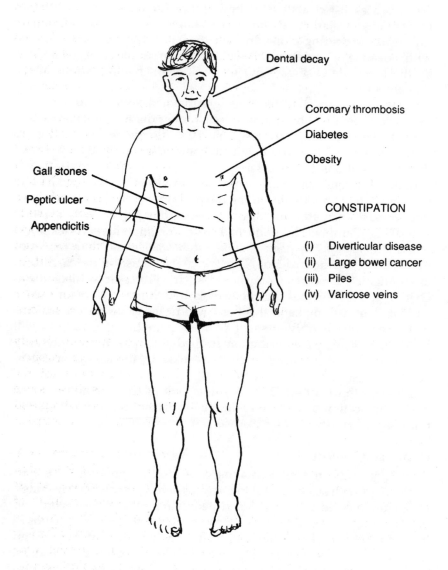

Dental decay

Coronary thrombosis

Diabetes

Obesity

Gall stones

Peptic ulcer

Appendicitis

CONSTIPATION

(i)   Diverticular disease
(ii) Large bowel cancer
(iii) Piles
(iv) Varicose veins

Fig. 6: *T. L. Cleave's Neglected Concept*
Diseases caused by eating refined carbohydrates
(Source: author)

Denis Burkitt returned to London from Uganda, where for some twenty years he had worked, first as a surgeon in the colonial medical service and then, since 1964, as a member of the external staff of the British Medical Research Council. His name was well known throughout the academic world for his part in the discovery of a virus-induced cancer, common in young children in certain parts of Africa, in whom it often presented as an unsightly swelling of the neck or jaw. The cancer had been named 'Burkitt's Lymphoma'.

Denis Burkitt's work with the Medical Research Council was concerned with the geographic distribution of disease. Soon after his arrival at his research council's office in London a meeting between him and Peter Cleave was arranged by Sir Richard Doll. Burkitt later wrote in his book, *Don't Forget Fibre in Your Diet*, 'meeting Captain Cleave was one of the most important occasions in my professional life. Background patterns of disease in the third world enabled me to recognise instantly the undeniable truth and logic of his ideas. I also had unique opportunities through medical contacts in most of Africa and Asia to confirm or deny statements he had made, and as will be shown later in this book, the mass of opinion endorsed his conclusions. Most of the medical profession at this time viewed Captain Cleave's ideas with scepticism, and consequently his evidence was rejected without proper consideration.'[6]

Denis Burkitt, an enthusiastic, versatile and witty speaker, already in demand worldwide as a lecturer on his African cancer research, realised the enormous importance of Cleave's discoveries for the future health of nations. With customary zeal, he used his considerable gifts as a communicator to spread Cleave's teaching. His writings and lectures in the 1970s and 80s stimulated renewed interest in nutrition among doctors and public.

Cleave's final book, *The Saccharine Disease*, published in 1974, achieved a wide readership. In 1976 he was elected to the fellowship of the Royal College of Physicians and, in 1979, his work was at last given public recognition by the award from the Royal Institute of Public Health and Hygiene of the Harben gold medal. This award is given for outstanding discoveries in the promotion of public health; previous recipients include Lister, Pasteur and Fleming. At the same ceremony held at the Haslar Royal Naval Hospital in Portsmouth, Cleave was also awarded the Gilbert Blane Medal, given by the royal colleges for work in promoting health in the Royal Navy.

---

6. D. Burkitt, *Don't Forget Fibre in Your Diet* (Martin Dentz, 1979), p. 12

Conflict of Opinions

At last, it seemed, Cleave's teaching was to be implemented and his unique contribution to medical thought recognised; but in the years that followed this did not happen; in spite of professional acclamation expressed in these awards, Cleave's work is now seldom mentioned by those in authority who concern themselves with the nation's health. A recent report by the Committee on Medical Aspects of Food Policy on Dietary Sugar and Human Disease[7] made no reference at all to Cleave's research. One reason for this strange neglect was anticipated by Cleave's penetrating observation that scientists, conditioned to wrestling with complex problems, often cannot understand simple concepts nor recognise their importance.

The understanding of the full significance of the saccharine disease became blurred when those who followed Cleave, especially Denis Burkitt, talked only of dietary fibre and excluded the far more import-ant effects of overconsumption. Cleave became increasingly irritated when it seemed that Burkitt sought to assume the role of maestro, with Cleave as novice, and to be bent on altering out of all recognition the material which he, Cleave, had so painstakingly gathered. This was particularly true when Burkitt dismissed sugar consumption as the cause of coronary thrombosis and joined those who, contrary to Cleave, blamed animal fat. 'Maps made by early navigators invariably have been enormously modified by subsequent cartographers, but this detracts nothing from the contribution from the original discovery',[8] wrote Burkitt; but Cleave was convinced that his thesis embraced fundamental biological truths which simply could not be 'enormously modified'. A work of classic dimensions cannot be enormously modi-fied without being spoilt, and when Burkitt played down the mechan-ism of overconsumption, Cleave felt like an artist whose canvas was being ruined by someone who did not really understand the original. The details of the differences in this debate need not concern us here, but I hope to enlarge on 'overconsumption' when discussing diabetes in a later chapter.

These differences do, however, underline what I tried to emphasise in my introduction, that conflicts are inevitable when scientific proof of a nutritional theory will always be beyond human reach. Human beings cannot be caged like laboratory animals and laboratory feeding experiments are not always applicable to humans; we have to fall back on guesswork. According to Cleave, we will guess correctly only

---

7. Department of Health, *Dietary Sugars and Human Disease*, No. 37 (London, HMSO, 1989)
8. D. Burkitt, *Don't Forget Fibre in Your Diet* (Martin Dentz, 1979), p. 13

if we understand nature's laws, and the perfect adaptation of human beings to their food supply as it occurs in nature. He often said to me, 'I may be wrong, and you may be wrong, but one thing is certain – nature is never wrong.'

Perfection of evolution

Varicose veins such as those which troubled Mrs McBeen are extremely common in Britain. Textbooks blame congenital weakness of the veins and man's upright posture as part of the cause. They thus suggest that 'nature' has made a mistake and that the human body has been, in a substantial minority of people, constructed wrongly. In Cleave's philosophy this is absurd. Certain Africans still living according to tribal traditions have been found to be virtually free of varicose veins. This same racial stock, when transplanted to America, in the course of time develops varicose veins on the same scale as do white Americans.

As an example of evolutionary perfection, I am sure that Cleave would point to the white mountain hare, sitting motionless on the snow as we climbed on our way to High Ridge Farm. Here is one of nature's miracles; as winter brings its covering of white on the moors, the grey-brown fur of the hare turns white – a perfect camouflage from the soaring eagle. This happens without the help of human intelligence; it is done by the wisdom of creation. Is it conceivable that nature, evolution, creation or any term the reader may wish to use, would perform this miracle in the mountain hare and yet make such a botch of human adaptation that millions of human beings were made lame or uncomfortable because their veins were not working properly?

If we agree that varicose veins are not caused by any fault of nature, and that their cause, according to Cleave's thesis, is simply due to lack of dietary fibre in modern diets, we must examine in the next chapter how this comes about.

8 Maggie and her Constipation

The emotional response to night-time calls passes through several well-defined phases. The first phase attempts to suppress feelings of considerable anger and hostility towards the caller, especially when the message seems to be vague and the need for a visit doubtful. These feelings accompany the fumbling for suitable clothes to put on over one's pyjamas. Return to full waking consciousness brings an effort to remember previous encounters with the patient and the possible requirements for this particular emergency. By the time one is on the way to the garage a reasonable state of alertness has been established, the worst of the pain is over, and there may even be a sense of anticipation for the challenge which lies ahead. Changing seasons give differing flavours to every emergency night call.

On this occasion, when her mother phoned at about 4 a.m. to say that Maggie, now aged around nineteen, had a 'sair belly' and that appendicitis was feared, February had come with bitter weather. There had been some snow on the previous day; more had fallen in the night, and it was clear that I would have to walk most of the way up the hill road to Maggie's cottage. As I feared, the car stuck as soon as I turned off the main road and attempted to drive up the hill. The cold was perishing, freezing the nostrils with each inward breath. But there has not been much drifting with this fall, so nowhere was the snow deep enough to come over my gumboots, and although progress was slow and laborious it might have been worse.

I had put on my warmest coat for the journey, at that time my old army overcoat. As I plodded along in the biting cold, carrying my bag, slipping and stumbling, I saw myself identified, as in a dream, with Napoleon's straggling soldiers as they retreated from Moscow. The sense of misery was further enhanced by the certainty, which had only been a suspicion as I set out, that my throat was sore and I was about to catch the flu-like illness which was then prevalent. The night was clear but there was no moon, so I had to use my torch to follow the line of the path down the bank of a small glen and over the footbridge which led to the cottage.

Maggie looked remarkably well, with pulse rate and temperature normal. Examination failed to reveal any convincing signs of appendicitis, but her pelvic colon was obviously heavily loaded and rectal examination was not really possible because it was packed solid with faeces. In short, Maggie was dreadfully constipated. I gave my diagnosis and suggested that with the dawn we would arrange for her to be admitted to the cottage hospital for observation and a wash out. The relief of the patient and of her parents at the diagnosis, and expressions of gratitude for the visit, banished all earlier feelings of resentment. 'You'll have a cup of tea, Doctor?' The tea, taken by the blazing fire, was comforting. Maggie's father was an estate handyman and seemed to spend all his time cutting logs, which were beautifully stacked round the cottage. Soon, when he retired, the family would move to the village in the valley below. The cottage would be renovated for the reception of summer visitors.

Maggie's predicament is of great importance to our understanding of the cause of varicose veins. Examples of similar extreme degrees of constipation are not at all uncommon; they are, I believe, the tip of the iceberg of a condition which in Scotland at any rate is near universal. 'Iceberg' is probably an apt comparison, in that the solid state of ice contrasts with the fluidity of the water from which it is derived. Maggie's colon was packed with relatively hard faecal matter – an abnormal or unnatural state of affairs, brought about by her diet, woefully deficient in many essential constituents, of which fibre is one of the most important.

The motions of people eating food from which fibre has not been removed by refining tend to be soft and bulky; they pass easily, often more than once daily. A constipated colon may permit the daily passage of hard motion, but it is still constipated; a history of daily bowel movement, therefore, is not always indicative of the unconstipated state, it may merely indicate daily overflow.[1]

As the large trunk veins from the legs pass up through the pelvis on their way to the heart, they lie close behind certain segments of the large bowel. When the latter is constantly loaded with hard, solid matter, pressure is exerted on the walls of the underlying veins; this abnormal pressure partly impedes the flow of blood upwards to the

1. A. R. P. Walker, 'Diet, bowel mobility, faeces composition and colon cancer', *South African Medical Journal* (April 1971), pp. 377–79

heart. Raised pressure within the veins below the point of obstruction stretches the valves, which become incompetent; so the veins, through time, develop the swollen, tortuous pattern which we know as the deformities of varicose veins.[2]

The colon-vein contact is closer on the left side than on the right, hence the more frequent occurrence of varicose veins and varicose ulcer on the left leg. It is crucial to Cleave's concept to reject utterly the thought that the fault lies in the structure of the human body. The fault, as he repeats again and again, is not in the way the human body is built, but in how it is used. Some individuals are so made that the abnormal pressures do not occur. Not every constipated person will suffer from varicose veins; but people who do not consume refined, fibre-depleted food do not suffer from varicose veins at all. This has been convincingly demonstrated in certain parts of Africa. Thanks to his contacts with medical colleagues in Uganda, Zululand and Nigeria, Cleave was able to confirm from the evidence of hospital statistics and from certain careful medical surveys of rural populations that varicose veins simply did not occur in tribal-living Africans.[3] There is no question of these records being unreliable.[4] Nor is there any doubt that Africans living in America, of the same racial stock as those who are free from varicose veins, suffer from this condition on the same scale as do white Americans.

In their tribal lands most of those Africans eat large quantities of unrefined maize meal; the amount of dietary fibre from this source is far higher than from the refined food of the West. The motions produced on this high-fibre diet are soft, bulky and easily passed without straining. Another feature of the high-fibre regime is the speed with which the bowel contents complete the passage from stomach to evacuation. Many studies have now been done, using markers to time the speed of bowel passage (transit time) in various populations. The data (for which see Table 1) taken from a paper by D. P. Burkitt, A. R. P. Walker and N. S. Painter give an extreme example of the contrast in bowel function between rural Africans and British naval ratings and their wives.

---

2. T. L. Cleave, *On the Causation of Varicose Veins* (Bristol, John Wright, 1960)
3. T. L. Cleave, *The Saccharine Disease* (Bristol, John Wright, 1974), p. 45
4. H. Dodd, 'The Cause, Prevention and Arrest of Varicose Veins', *The Lancet*, 7363, vol. 2 (1964) pp. 809–11

Table 1: *Effect of dietary fibre on stools and transit times*

Subjects	Number	Country	Race	Mean transit time: hours	Mean weight of stool passed: gm.
Naval ratings and wives	15	UK	White	83.4	104
Rural villagers	15	Uganda	African	33.5	470

Source: *The Lancet*, 7792, vol. 2 (1972), pp. 1408–11

Africans who eat diets heavily dependent on refined maize may be prone to nutritional deficiencies and to infections, as this diet is not always a balanced one, but they do not suffer from those western diseases associated with constipation – varicose veins, diverticular disease and colon (or large bowel) cancer.

The spread of processed foods

As trade routes, food processing technology and cash economies spread ever further throughout the continents of the world, the contrast in bowel function and disease patterns between 'primitives' and Europeans is likely to diminish; as they change from home-pounded maize meal to white bread, Africans will become more constipated and prone to the diseases mentioned above.

On our visit in 1985 to Dr Halley Stott, founder of the Valley Trust in Natal,[5] I learned that Zulu farmers were selling their maize harvests for cash and then using their earnings to purchase *refined* maize flour for their own consumption. The same change in trading habits has spread throughout the world as farmers or crofters use the earnings from the sale of their products for the purchase of imported processed foods. No longer do they see their own land as the main source of their nourishment.

Health in rural Scotland

In the opening decades of the nineteenth century it is probable that freedom from non-infective diseases, some of which we have discussed in this chapter, gave a measure of health and vigour to middle-aged and elderly rural Scots, which has since been lost. The agricultural improvements of the eighteenth century had by that time spread to the Highlands from England and from the Scottish lowlands; at the same time new railway and road networks were not yet in place to make possible the import of large quantities of processed foods, including white flour and sugar.

5. B. S. Young, 'The Valley Trust', *Canadian Geographical Journal* (June 1965)

A Doctor in the Wilderness

In her book, *The Good Scots Diet*,[6] Maisie Steven analyses the diet of a male agricultural worker at the end of the eighteenth century. It featured oatmeal, barley, potatoes, turnips, kale, cheese, butter, milk and ale; these foods nourished a rural population which seems to have been long-lived and healthy; on that fibre-rich food we can be confident that they did not suffer from constipation and its complications. Mrs Steven gives the following extract from the Statistical Account of 1791–99 for the parish of Fortingall, west of Aberfeldy. 'In general the people are pretty long-lived. Many are between 80 and 90; some between 90 and 100; a few live beyond that age. There is, at present, a gentleman living and still healthy and strong aged 103 ... the present incumbent likewise knew, about 30 years ago, one Donald Cameron, who lived, it was credibly asserted, to the amazing age of 127'.[7]

The author of this information, 'the present incumbent', was, of course, the Presbyterian parish minister of Fortingall, who with his fellow ministers throughout Scotland were cajoled by Sir John Sinclair to respond to a list of 160 queries which would enable the government 'not only to assess its current state but to prepare for a better future ... their reports provide us today with an incomparable view of Scotland two centuries ago, through the sharp eyes and the often sharp words of men who knew their localities very well indeed'.[8]

That charming word-picture of nineteenth-century life in 'Drumtochty', a Perthshire village not far from here, *Beside the Bonny Briar Bush*,[9] gives this account of longevity in those days:

Drumtochty was accustomed to break every law of health, except wholesome food and fresh air, and yet had reduced the Psalmist's further limit to an average life-rate ... The ordinary course of life, with fine air and contented minds, was to do a full share of work until 70, and then to look after 'orra' jobs well into the 80s and to 'slip awa' within sight of 90. Persons of about 90 were understood to be acquitting themselves with credit, and assumed airs of authority, brushing aside the opinions of 70 as immature, and confirming their conclusions with illustrations drawn from the end of the last century.

6. Maisie Steven, *The Good Scots Diet: What Happened to It?* (Aberdeen University Press, 1985)
7. *The Statistical Account of Scotland*, vol. 12, North West Perthshire, 1791–1799 (Edinburgh, Blackwoods)
8. *Ibid.*, p. iii
9. Ian McLaren, *Beside the Bonnie Briar Bush* (London, Hodder & Stoughton, 1894), pp. 229–30

In fact, *on average*, we appear to be living longer than did our forebears a hundred and fifty years ago; this is partly because infections, especially tuberculosis, no longer take their toll in infancy, youth or middle age; improved housing with central heating probably helps to keep elderly folk alive; so do the advances in medical care; but I wonder if the growing army of present-day citizens in their seventies and eighties can match the physical performance of elderly rustics as described above.

The dawn of a new age

The Second Statistical Account of 1845[10] gives the first warning of the revolution which, in the course of the next one hundred years or so, was to change out of all recognition the food and the way of life of the Scottish highlander. The parish minister of Kenmore, the Revd David Duff, in writing of the great improvements in agriculture and food production which had taken place in the preceding fifty years, stated:

> Irish-like, indeed, we use a vast deal of potatoes, but we manage to season these roots with a due mixture of beef, mutton, and pork; not to speak of the milk, cheese and butter with which we are supplied from our dairies or the higher dainties of tea and sugar . . . Independently of what many families import themselves there are, within the parish, for the convenience of the public, ten small retail shops . . . And as if all this were not enough, two rival bakers from Aberfeldie penetrate, twice a week upon an average, a considerable way into the parish with well stored carts to supplant our oaten cakes by the substitution of the luxury of wheaten bread.

The enterprising bakers with their white flour products were the first trickle of a flood of manufactured foods which were to replace local produce as the nourishment of the Scottish highlander. A full understanding of the condition of my patient, Maggie's, bowels, and those of the constipated thousands like her, is not possible without taking into account this history of trading patterns. The process was hastened here from 1867 when the first train pulled into Aberfeldy's new station; cheap manufactured food – white flour, sugar, margarine – could now be easily distributed far and wide, as could relatively cheap mass-produced clothes. The days of the rural weavers, cobblers, tanners

---

10. *The Second Statistical Account*, 1845 (Edinburgh, Blackwoods)

and flax dressers were numbered; so were the days of the millers and of many of the farmers who served them.

Home baking

Now that the new baking materials were available to them, hardworking housewives, proud of their baking prowess, hastened the change of diet in their families. The traditional Scottish high tea became a feast of starch and sugar, wherein the course of something cooked was followed by piles of scones, cakes and cookies; as kail yards became fewer, vegetables increasingly came out of cans. The very friendliness and hospitality of the country people added to the load of refined carbohydrate; the kindly cup of tea (usually heavily sweetened) offered as a symbol of welcome was always accompanied by cake or scones. To refuse a piece of mother's cake might be seen as an affront! What a pity that we did not accept the oriental custom that tea should be savoured for its own sake without having to consume starch or sugar!

As I drove home through the snow-bound village below Maggie's house I passed a row of cottages, one of which was due for a visit tomorrow (really today, already 5.30 a.m.). The patient was Mr Black whose bowels displayed the end result of a lifetime of constipation – widespread diverticular disease, the complications of which I will not detail here; suffice it to say that they had involved hours of surgical and medical care in hospital and had made his declining years a misery. Thanks to the research of Dr N. S. Painter,[11] the way in which constipation causes this condition is now well understood, as is its prevention. But however much I urge Maggie's family to eat wholewheat bread instead of white and to take salads, fruits and vegetables, I doubt if I will have much success; she will much prefer to take one of the popular laxatives and to continue eating the starch and sugar to which she is addicted.

11. T. L. Cleave, G. D. Campbell and N. S. Painter, *Diabetes, Coronary Thrombosis and the Saccharine Disease* (Bristol, John Wright, 1966), chapter 9

9 A Case of Cancer

December 1956 (diary entry):

Have just been down the street to see Mrs Smith, and have given her her nightly heroin; she can't be without it for she is dying of abdominal cancer. A good, capable and brave woman. What can I do? Nothing to halt the course of the disease. I know that God did not intend that human beings should rot away with this terrible disease. I say to myself that I must do something to teach people what I am beginning to realise is the right way of prevention. It is terrible at this time of Christmas to visit a patient such as this, wasting away in front of their families, while we as doctors are powerless. Is there something far wrong with present cancer research? It seems directed to trying to eradicate established disease instead of looking broadly at the problem as a whole.

As long ago as 1922, in a lecture entitled 'Faulty food in relation to gastro-intestinal disease', McCarrison told how in his early years in India he worked as doctor to certain isolated Himalayan peoples. Among these tribes, of whom the Hunzas were outstanding in health and vitality, in the nine years he lived and worked among them, he saw not a single case of duodenal ulcer, appendicitis or cancer. The absence of abdominal complaints among these healthy, long-lived tribesmen was, McCarrison observed, in marked contrast to the high incidence of various forms of indigestion and intestinal disease among British people, and especially to 'the alarming increase of cancer among town dwellers . . . due in the main to the increasing prevalence of gastro-intestinal cancer.'[1]

McCarrison found his explanation for the contrast between the

---

1. R. McCarrison, 'Faulty food in relation to gastro-intestinal disease', *Journal of the American Medical Association*, 89, vol. 1 (1922), pp. 1–9

widespread gastro-intestinal disease in the West and the abdominal health of the Himalayan tribesmen in the following four circumstances:

1. Infants are reared as nature intended them to be reared – at the breast.
2. People live on the unsophisticated foods of nature; milk, eggs, grains, fruits and vegetables. I don't suppose that one in every thousand of them has ever seen a tinned salmon, a chocolate or a patent infant food, nor that as much sugar is imported into their country in a year as is used in a modest-sized hotel of this city in a single day.
3. Their religion prohibits alcohol and, although they do not in this respect always lead a strictly religious life, nevertheless they are an eminently teetotal race.
4. Their manner of life requires vigorous exercise of their bodies.

Let us look at McCarrison's 'four circumstances' in the light of British habits to-day:

1) *Breast feeding*. A recent survey[2] found that only 51 per cent of British mothers fed their infants at the breast for as long as two weeks and a mere 26 per cent for four weeks or more.

2) *Unsophisticated foods of nature*. The four decades since the end of World War II have seen a remarkable growth in Britain of the sale and consumption of what are termed 'convenience foods' – pre-cooked, canned or frozen foods, which are essential in households where both parents are working. Fresh food, or freshly cooked food, cannot appear on the family table without someone spending more time in the kitchen than is required for merely warming up the contents of tin or packet. I do not know how this difficulty is to be resolved in an age when women, even women with young children, find it essential to have a job outside the home, and when they are encouraged to regard the kitchen as a place of drudgery (see Appendix I).

Milk and eggs are placed at the top of McCarrison's list of health-giving foods, a priority which is now contradicted by modern teaching to the effect that dairy food and eggs, because of their fat content, will damage our hearts. The evidence for such an extraordinary reversal

---

2. HMSO Social Survey Division, 'Infant Feeding 1985'

of previously accepted belief is totally unconvincing and will be discussed in a later chapter.

We have already discussed the degradation of wheat grains to produce white flour for modern milling; the grains of oats, traditionally Scotland's staple cereal, are not now our standard breakfast food; porridge has been widely replaced by a variety of sweetened, highly processed products. As for fruit and vegetables, here again in Scotland consumption is abysmally low, probably the lowest in Europe. Visitors from England and beyond to rural Scotland should find people on the whole friendly and the scenery the most magnificent in the world, but they will often search in vain, even in the height of summer, for a really fresh lettuce, cabbage or carrot, or a generous helping of fresh garden beans or peas. Such fruit as can be found in the shops will be expensive. The reason for this lack of fresh fruits and vegetables is partly climatic; our northern growing season is shorter than in the south, and apart from favoured lowland areas, apples, pears and similar fruits do not always crop well. But the west coast is washed by the Gulf Stream and, at sea level, enjoys mild winters. The magnificent vegetable garden at Poolewe in Ross-shire could, if enough people had the energy and the will, be emulated elsewhere. In our own Aberfeldy garden, a most inhospitable stony hillock in north Perthshire, we grow some 1,300 lb of vegetables and soft fruit annually.[3] We seldom go to the shops for vegetables.

Official household surveys of food consumption fully confirm the experience of visitors searching for fresh vegetables and salads in Scotland. Fig. 7 taken from the 1966 MAFF survey,[4] shows the weekly consumption of various foods in ounces per week per person in Scotland compared with southeast England. The extraordinarily low intake of fresh fruits and vegetables in Scotland is obvious, and twenty years later the surveys still show this unfortunate deficiency. Similar figures in both regions for 'sugar and preserves' might seem to contradict the opinion repeatedly stressed here that Scotland's poor health is due to a higher intake of refined carbohydrate foods. But as home cooking has declined in the last thirty years, and as the purchase by households of manufactured foods has increased, 60 per cent of sugar is now consumed as an additive to processed foods. So when the sugar content of buns, cakes and sweet biscuits is taken into account, the higher

3. W. W. Yellowlees, 'Ill fares the land', *Journal of the Royal College of General Practitioners*, vol. 29 (1979), pp. 7–21
4. Ministry of Agriculture, Fisheries and Food, Household Food Consumption and Expenditure (HMSO 1966)

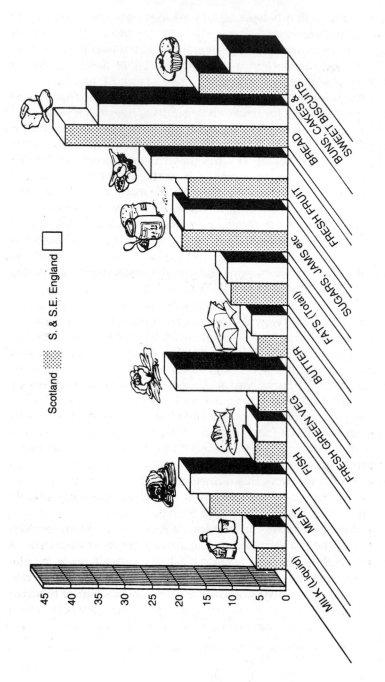

Fig. 7: *Household food consumption*
(Source: Ministry of Agriculture and Food, HMSO, 1966)

sugar consumption in Scotland is obvious. National food surveys do not assess confectionery or soft drinks. Some years ago, in answer to my queries about regional differences in the consumption of sweets, I was told by a representative of a well-known confectionery firm that no data were available on this subject.

Dependence on foods made from white flour laced with sugar in place of fresh fruits and vegetables is a feature of life in the north and northwest of England, as well as in Scotland.[5] It is also a feature of the eating habits of the lower income groups[6] who consume far more of these degraded foods than do social class I. The higher death rates among (a) the Scots, (b) the people of northwest England and (c) the lower income groups, seem therefore to confirm McCarrison's conclusions that of all factors that make for health, sound nutrition is the most important. A similar pattern emerges from the finding of the breast feeding survey mentioned above, that among social classes I and II and in the southeast of England, mothers were more likely to feed their infants at the breast than those in social class V and in the north.

3) *Alcohol.* The malt sugar present in beer is a form of refined carbo-hydrate, a fact which helps to explain why beer-drinking young men, although they are often engaged in work involving much muscular activity, yet through time develop unsightly protuberant bellies; their consumption of two, three, four or more pints of this beverage daily adds to the total load of refined carbohydrate.

As to wine, 'Wine that maketh glad the heart of man' (Psalm 104, verse 15), or again

Inflaming wine pernicious to mankind,
Unnerves the limbs and dulls the noble mind
(Pope's translation of Homer's *Iliad*);

readers can choose which of the above quotations they prefer. The damage to human health caused by the excessive alcohol intake of the addict is well documented, and will not be dwelt on here. The dying patient mentioned in my diary did not drink alcohol, nor did she smoke. McCarrison does not tell us if the Hunzas smoked tobacco; in his day lung cancer was a rare cause of death, and the link between

5. *Ibid.*
6. H. Clayton, *The Times*, 18 April, 1978

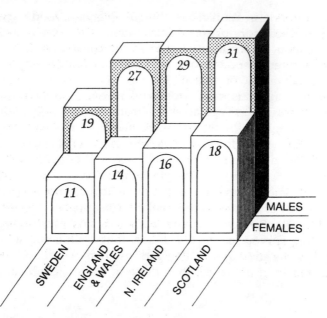

Fig. 8: *Percentage of persons aged 44 years who will not survive to age 65 years in Sweden and in the UK. (1972 death rates)*
(Source: Prevention and Health, *DHSS, HMSO, 1976)*

heavy cigarette smoking and various diseases had not yet been observed.

4) Exercise. I do not intend to dwell on McCarrison's fourth circumstance which he believed was necessary for health – plenty of exercise – but would commend to readers the views of Dr Kenneth Vickery, who devotes a chapter of his book, *Choose Health, Choose Life*, to a discussion on the virtues of regular exercise and the dangers of the modern craze for jogging.[7]

In discussing the first three of McCarrison's headings I hope that the answer is emerging to the cry of distress entered in my diary of 1956, as I came from a visit to a patient dying from spreading abdominal cancer. If the types of cancer common in the west are to be prevented, changes in our dietary habits are essential. But although the changes as outlined by Cleave and McCarrison are simple, immense

7. Kenneth Vickery, *Choose Health, Choose Life* (Eastbourne, Kingsway Publications, 1986)

difficulties stand in the way of change. Consumers are already so confused and bored by the unceasing torrent of advice, information and propaganda about diet, that many wish to hear no more. But our plight is serious, especially in Scotland, where more people die between the ages of 45 and 65 than in other parts of the United Kingdom. The comparison with Sweden is dismal indeed (see fig. 8). Cancer accounts for about 23 per cent of all deaths in Scotland.

In the Aberfeldy practice, before I retired in 1981, we diagnosed on average seventeen new cases of cancer every year, of which colon cancer was the most common. From 1 January 1975 until 31 December 1981, twenty-seven new cases of this form of cancer were diagnosed here. Twenty-seven cases in seven years in the 3,600 people living in a Highland glen is in stark contrast to McCarrison's failure in nine years to discover one single case among 13,000 inhabitants of the Hunza valley.

10 More on Cancer

Many scientists would dismiss McCarrison's failure to record a single case of cancer among Himalayan tribesmen as of no consequence; they would say that no reliance can be placed on 'anecdotal' evidence from a primitive country devoid of written medical records. But McCarrison was a conscientious scientist whose observations were always made with care and objectivity. He was not given to exaggeration, and worked as a doctor among these people for nine years. Other travellers confirmed his description of the Hunzas as a people who enjoyed remarkable freedom from disease.

The absence of colonic cancer among isolated peoples having no access to modern foods has now been recorded repeatedly in other parts of the world.[1] The association of this form of cancer with constipation is widely agreed, but the exact mechanism which gives rise to cancerous changes in the constipated bowel is not as well understood as is the way in which constipation causes varicose veins, haemorrhoids or diverticular disease.

Consumption of saturated fat has been blamed as a cause of colon and breast cancer.[2] (At present it is fashionable to blame dietary fat as the cause of many modern diseases.) Cleave, however, holds that refined sugar, consumed in quantities of about 100 lb. per annum, now customary in the West, brings about tremendous proliferation of unwanted bacteria, especially E. coli in the colon; such unnatural bacterial growth in turn produces abnormal faecal breakdown products, some of which may be carcinogenic. The offensive smell typical of stools passed by people whose food contains much refined sugar is, according to this analysis, abnormal and may be taken as a sign that

---

1 H. C. Trowell and D. P. Burkitt, *Western Diseases: Their Emergence and Prevention* (London, Edward Arnold, 1981), p. 39
2. *Ibid.*, p. 102

intestinal toxaemia – a thing ridiculed by teachers of my generation – does indeed exist.

We cannot leave the discussion of cancer and its causes without touching briefly on the following: 1. Carcinogens. 2. Vitamin deficiency. 3. Organically grown food. 4. Cholesterol-lowering regimes.

1. Carcinogens

Repeated exposure to certain substances induce the cellular changes of cancer; of these the carcinogen most prominent in recent decades is benzpyrene, found in the tar and smoke of tobacco; year by year evidence accumulates which demonstrates that smokers are more likely to suffer from other cancers in addition to cancer of the lungs: the latest is leukemia.[3]

Cigarette smoking is rightfully condemned as a harmful, dangerous habit, but writers on this subject tend to ignore the fact that populations with the highest death rates from lung cancer do not always have the highest consumption of tobacco. Quoting from WHO statistics, Arthur and Margaret Wynn remind us that in the Netherlands, Switzerland, West Germany and Japan, people consume more tobacco per head of the population than in the United Kingdom, but suffer far less from lung cancer.[4] For instance, in 1973, Scotsmen aged between 45 and 54 died from lung cancer at a rate of 94 per 100,000 of the population. For the same age group in Japan the rate was 13, a sevenfold difference. Eskimos are also heavy smokers, but on their traditional diet have a very low or zero incidence of all forms of cancer.[5] Dr Hugh Sinclair and others believe that their immunity is due to the large quantities of essential fatty acids in the marine fats which they eat.[6]

All this suggests that populations like the Scots who suffer severely from cancer may simply be showing lower resistance to this disease. As we have seen, McCarrison demonstrated that of all factors that make for health, and therefore for sound resistance or defence against the various toxic agents which beset us, perfect nutrition was by far the most important. In other words, people subsisting on health-giving foods will more often successfully defend themselves against carcinogens than those whose food is defective. But, as with bacteria

3. Nicholas Wald, 'Smoking and leukaemia', *BMJ*, 6649, vol. 297, p. 628
4. M. Wynne and A. Wynne, *Prevention of Handicap and the Health of Women* (London, Routledge and Kegan Paul, 1979), pp. 86–8
5. V. Steffanson, *Cancer: Disease of Civilisation?* (New York, Hill and Wrang, 1960)
6. H. M. Sinclair, 'Fish oil and plasma fibrinogen', *BMJ*, 6648, vol. 297, p. 615 (1988)

or viruses, overwhelming doses of carcinogen may defeat the strongest defences.

The mushroom growth of the chemical industry during and since World War II has released into our environment an awesome tonnage of toxic materials which contaminate our air, food and water on a scale not easily measured; nor will it ever be within our scientific skills to know how many of these newer chemicals, acting alone or in combination with others, are carcinogenic.

One estimate of our dependence on artificial food additives gives an average consumption of 10 grams daily.[7] The total number of artificial food additives now appears to be around 3,500. They are divided into the following sections: preservatives, colours, anti-oxidants, emulsifiers, stabilisers, sweeteners, solvents, mineral hydrocarbons and miscellaneous.[8] Of this cocktail 5 per cent consists of colouring agents, and sixteen of them are manufactured from coal tar. Coal tar dyes are 'preferred in the food industry because they are more stable'.[9] Brightly coloured fizzy or soft drinks, beloved by children, owe their brilliance to these coal tar derivatives; one of these, the red dye given the European (E) number 123, aramanth, has been banned in the USA and the former USSR because tests suggested a link between ingestion of the dye and cancer and birth defects in laboratory rats. It is widely used in food and drink in the UK.

One possible indicator of the overdosage of toxic materials in which the British people are now drenched is the gradual increase in incidence and death rates over the last three decades from asthma. The authors of a review of this worrying phenomenon concluded as follows:

We can only speculate that our response mechanism to airborne irritants is being modified gradually by dietary factors, by disease processes or by other factors that we do not understand; alternatively contamination of the environment by potential irritants (new or existing) may have increased. The patterns of increase for both asthma and hay fever are similar, suggesting a common explanatory factor.[10]

7. Sheila Bingham, *Food and Nutrition: The Everyman Companion* (London, J. M. Dent & Son, 1987), p. 1
8. *Ibid.*, p. 70
9. *Ibid.*, p. 70
10. D. M. Fleming and D. L. Crombie, 'Prevalence of asthma and hay fever in England and Wales', *BMJ*, 6567, vol. 294, pp. 261–324

2. Vitamin deficiency

In a feeding trial in which he used monkeys, McCarrison found that when cereal food was heated in order to destroy all vitamins of the B group, widespread degenerative changes of the stomach and intestines were observed; one subject developed an early cancer of the stomach.[11] More recent evidence[12] has confirmed the protective role of vitamin-rich green or yellow vegetables against certain forms of cancer, and tests using laboratory animals have identified vitamins A and C as possessing this effect. The importance of vitamin C will be discussed in chapter 13.

3. Organically grown food

Beata Bishop, a London businesswoman, gives a vivid account[13] of how she was found in 1980 to be suffering from a malignant melanoma, one of the most lethal and quickest-spreading forms of skin cancer. The tumour on her lower leg was removed surgically by widespread resection requiring an extensive skin graft. Assurances that the cancer had been successfully removed and would not recur proved to be wrong when, about six months later, a hard lump appeared in her groin.

Horrified by the thought of another mutilating operation, she sought alternative treatment at a clinic in Mexico, where a strict dietary regime evolved by the late Dr Gerson is used as a treatment for patients with cancer, many of whom had not been cured by conventional surgery, radiotherapy or chemotherapy. The rationale of this treatment is to stimulate and encourage the body's own defences against cancer. This is done by a formidable programme of daily enemas and regular feeding with juices extracted from organically grown vegetables and fruits; a puree prepared from raw liver also featured in the dietary regime.

Ridicule and laughter would, I am sure, be the response of most orthodox medical scientists to this history. But one cannot laugh off the fact that the patient survived and was restored to normal health and well-being. Her secondary tumour did not spread, and when it was later removed under a local anaesthetic the cancer cells were seen to have been walled off by scar tissue which formed a protective capsule. It is surely wrong to dismiss all this as unsubstantiated rub-

11. H. M. Sinclair, *The Work of Sir Robert McCarrison*. (London, Faber, 1953), p. 198
12. H. C. Trowell and D. P. Burkitt, *Western Diseases: Their Emergence and Prevention* (London, Edward Arnold, 1981), p. 104
13. Beata Bishop, *A Time to Heal* (London, Severn House Publishers, 1985)

bish, without a careful study of the claims of success in cancer treatment at the Gerson clinic.

According to Ms Bishop, Dr Gerson placed great importance on the protective effect against cancer of organic produce. This claim is not new. The excessive use of soluble chemicals in agriculture can cause profound changes and imbalances in the soil, which in turn affect the availability to animals and man of minerals, some of which are essential components of enzyme systems. For instance, severe deficiency of copper and selenium have been demonstrated in animals grazing on crops grown in soil receiving repeated heavy applications of nitrogenous chemical fertilisers.[14] Such deficiencies appear to have increased greatly in the farmlands of western Scotland in the last twenty years.[15] Some studies have suggested that deficiencies of copper and selenium bring an increased susceptibility to cancer.[16]

In a series of laboratory feeding experiments, using pigeons and rats, McCarrison found that organically grown grains seemed to have superior nutritive qualities compared with grains grown with the use of chemical fertilisers.[17] The Hunzas, whose health and survival depended utterly on their own agriculture, returned all their wastes to the soil in the form of carefully made composts; a network of channels irrigated their terraced plots and every year the springtime thaw brought a bonus of mineral-bearing silt from melting glaciers.[18] McCarrison believed that the superior quality of organically grown crops was due to vitamin-like action, especially vitamins of the B group and vitamin A.

4. Cholesterol-lowering regimes

In 1978 a report was published of a large-scale European study carried out over five and a half years under the auspices of the WHO.[19] The study was designed to discover if heart attacks could be prevented by the use of a drug, Clofibrate, to lower blood cholesterol levels in a selected group of men. One alarming outcome of this trial, to be more fully discussed in chapter 18, was a marked increase in the incidence of cancer among subjects whose blood cholesterol had been successfully lowered. No one knows whether this was due to some unsuspected

14. Andre Voisin, *Soil, Grass and Cancer* (London, Crosby Lockwood, 1959)
15. J. Scott Park. Portnellan, Gartocharn, Dumbartonshire, 1988. Personal communication
16. W. C. Willett and M. J. Stamfer, 'Selenium and cancer', *BMJ*, 6648, vol. 297, p. 573 (1988)
17. R. McCarrison, 'The effect of manurial conditions on the nutritive and vitamin values of millet and wheat', *Indian Journal of Medical Research*, vol. 14 (1926), pp. 351–75
18. G. T. Wrench, *The Wheel of Health* (London, C. W. Daniel, 1938)
19. WHO, Committee of Principal Investigators, 'Cooperative trial', *British Heart Journal*, vol. 40 (1983), pp. 1069–1118

effect of the drug or to an unknown consequence of artificially manipulating cholesterol levels; nor is it clear whether lowering blood cholesterol by dietary measures might give the same unfortunate result. Studies on this subject are conflicting; cancer of the colon and rectum have been shown in one survey to be associated with lower levels of blood cholesterol,[20] and a recent very large study in America confirmed an inverse ratio between cancer deaths and blood cholesterol levels.[21] This last study was carried out over a long enough span of time to convince the authors that the lower cholesterol blood levels did not occur as a result of cancer, but seemed to be associated with its cause.

All this emphasises how little we know; but surely these findings should give pause to those who would have the whole population switch from butter to polyunsaturated margarine in the hope of preventing heart attacks by lowering blood cholesterol. Butter qualifies as an 'unsophisticated food of nature'; margarine does not. By 1922, the year in which McCarrison referred to the increase of gastro-intestinal cancer in the British urban population, margarine was for the first time being sold as a cheap form of dietary fat.[22]

What, then, is the final answer to the cry of anguish about cancer from a young GP as he emerged in 1956 from the house of a friend dying of that dread disease – carcinogens? Refined carbohydrates? Vitamins? Soil depletion? Too much saturated fat? The reader can be forgiven a sense of confusion. Not much light will be shed by studying the volumes of research papers which pour out annually on the subject of cancer. Indeed, to study them all is beyond the capacity of any single person. Whole departments have been created for researching one small facet of the disease. We may never understand in detail exactly how cancer cells emerge and grow, but we do know that unless our bodily defences are maintained with care, our fight against this disease will be in vain.

In keeping our defensive armour bright, McCarrison's philosophy is of immense importance. Health is wholeness, and that wholeness depends above all on fresh natural food, eaten in reasonable variety and grown on soil whose fertility is sustained by organic or biological methods. This teaching is extremely simple, but in the West we have largely departed from it. As we have seen, only a minority of mothers feed their infants at the breast, the virtue is processed out of our

20. G. Rose, H. Blackburn, A. Keys and others, 'Colon cancer and blood cholesterol', The Lancet, vol 1 (1974), pp. 181–3
21. A. Schatzkin, P. R. Taylor and others, 'Serum Cholesterol and Cancer in the NHANNES 1 Epidemiological Follow Up Study', The Lancet, 8554, vol. 2 (1988), pp. 298–301
22. W. Martin, 'Margarine, (not butter), the culprit', The Lancet, 8346, vol. 2 (1983), p. 407

food and our agriculture has become dependent on ever increasing applications of nitrogenous fertilisers and pesticides. Alcohol and tobacco loom large in our lives.

The case history to be recounted in the next chapter could only occur in a country where consumers and producers of food had lost their way. How sad that that country should be Scotland, once famed for the vigorous health of her people.

11   Scurvy on the Farm

It is unwise to go visiting the sick in angry mood and folly to display one's anger. The upshot is usually a missed diagnosis, often an outraged patient and, sometimes, deterioration beyond repair of that mysterious bond, the doctor-patient relationship.

But it was difficult on this occasion not to be angry. Had I not already in the course of a busy day twice passed the Haugh Farm road-end? And now, at the end of the day, when I had hoped for a precious hour in the greenhouse among the seed boxes, here was a message demanding a visit; typical, I thought, of the McToshes of the Haugh. The two middle-aged brothers, Dave and Willie, worked the place in their own haphazard fashion, growing mostly hay to feed their small herd of cattle.

Some years ago, regular visits to the farm had been necessary when Dave's crippled wife was still alive. Latterly, her increasing congestive heart failure had limited her domestic activities to stirring the soup or peeling the taties; eventually she had to agree to admission to a long-stay hospital, since when the brothers had done their own housekeeping. As I negotiated the twisting farm road, I recalled the scene which awaited me in the Mill Farm kitchen: in each corner of the room mounds of dusty newspapers and old clothes, the large kitchen table littered with the debris of past meals – crusts of bread, half-empty tins, grimy pots and pans. Under the table a brown hen used to crouch, her attitude of silent despair somehow in keeping with the surroundings.

A quick glance as I entered assured me that the scene had not changed except that the hen was not there. Willie McTosh was upstairs in bed; the evening light which filtered through a window grimed with dust and thick with cobwebs revealed chaos no less than in the kitchen.

My suppressed fury at being called up here at the end of the day was not calmed when Willie gave his complaint as a 'sair knee', the result of a trivial injury sustained about a week ago. Clothed in a flannel shirt, woollen vest and long underpants, he lay in a bed ungraced by any linen. The 'long johns' had obviously not been washed for a very long time; I could not face removing them at this late hour. The supposedly injured knee showed no sign of swelling, and the joint could be moved through a full range of movement, without pain. 'You've strained your knee, Willie,' I said.

'Just so, doctor,' he replied, 'just so.'

Willie was a quiet, simple chap. At the time of visits to his late sister-in-law he was usually hanging about the kitchen, eager for a 'crack' about the price of cattle or the state of the nation. Often on those occasions he thought up a complaint of his own which seldom seemed to have any basis apart from attention-seeking. Probably, I thought, he had got me up here because he wanted someone to talk to – his brother was inclined to be silent. So, fighting back my exasperation, I said, 'I'll send you some stuff to rub on, and in a day or two you'll be alright,' and prepared to go.

But then I paused, aware of a tinge of guilt which coloured my anger. Even in this light was his complexion, beneath farmyard grime, a bit greyer than usual? So I returned to the bed and, to atone for my hitherto inadequate examination, took off 2.5 cm. of venous blood. What a boon to visiting GPs is the new invention of disposable syringes and needles which gives us the means of rapid blood screening without the tedious, time-consuming business of boiling and autoclaving. When the laboratory is thirty miles away, if quick results are to be obtained an accurate haemoglobinmeter in the surgery is essential. Our newly purchased Grey Wedge photometer seemed to be the best instrument for the GP's work place.

Back in the surgery the efficiency of the method was painfully apparent; the pointer rested at 43 per cent (normal 80–100 per cent). Something was seriously amiss; I had wronged poor Willie! Too late to go back now, but next morning I hurried back to the farm and in the stronger light of day could see that Willie had indeed the unhealthy pallor of severe anaemia.

Routine examination of heart and lungs revealed no abnormality, but the 'long johns' would have to be tackled. When they were finally removed the appearance of Willie's legs would have caused a medical photographer to rush for his camera. Vast purple, blue and violet patches spread from mid-thigh to mid-calf on the left side and to a lesser extent on the right. Over his back and abdomen were other patches of discolouration, all due to ecchymoses (bleeding under the skin). Another large blotch of spreading blue had developed at the site of last night's venipuncture.

A case of profound anaemia and widespread subcutaneous bleeding would, I knew, be welcomed by the consultant physicians at Perth, but I felt confident that the kitchen table was the key to the diagnosis, so admitted Willie to the cottage hospital and gave him a course of multi-vitamin injections and a diet rich in orange juice. In a few weeks he recovered completely.

Willie was suffering from scurvy, caused by deficiency in his diet of ascorbic acid or vitamin C, a deficiency which, had it continued, would have killed him. Two features of his case are of importance for the theme of this book; simplicity and the implications of widespread, sub-clinical deficiency.

1. Simplicity

Here is a disease, potentially fatal, one, moreover, having widespread bodily and mental manifestations, the cause of which is supremely simple. The signs and symptoms of scurvy include lassitude and depression, bleeding gums, loss of teeth, painful joints, the breaking down of old scars and the failure of wounds to heal – all for want of fresh food, particularly fruits and vegetables.

In 1753 James Lind, an Edinburgh graduate and naval surgeon, demonstrated clearly[1] that scurvy, which at that time was decimating the crews of far-voyaging sailing ships, could be prevented when the standard seafaring ration of pickled meat and ship's biscuits was supplemented by citrus fruits or their juices. This life-saving discovery was rejected by the eighteenth-century physicians whose minds were in the grip of the orthodoxy of their time. To them cures could only be effected by medicines concocted according to elaborate prescriptions, the ingredients of which bore the stamp of witchcraft. 'Some persons', declared the exasperated Lind, 'cannot be brought to believe that a disease, so fatal and so dreadful, can be cured or prevented by such easy means. They would have more faith in an elaborate composition dignified with the title of an "anti-scorbutic elixir" or the like!'[2]

Some fifty years were to pass, following the publication by Lind of his discovery, before a daily issue of lemon juice was adopted by the navy. James Lind's exasperation is echoed today by those of us who

1. B. Inglis, *A History of Medicine* (London, Weidenfeld and Nicolson, 1965), pp. 114–15
2. *Ibid*

find it hard to understand why the teaching of another Royal Naval surgeon, T. L. Cleave, is totally neglected by medical scientists. The same exasperation on a broader front is justified by the neglect of the work of Sir Robert McCarrison. It is now more than fifty years since he gave the summing-up of his life's work in three Canton lectures later published in book form.

In recent years there has certainly been a widespread stirring of interest in the role of nutrition in the cause and prevention of disease. But neither the medical profession nor those who run the so-called Health Service can bring themselves to believe that the 'easy means' of simple dietary change could transform the health of the nation.

2. The tip of another iceberg

I will be severely criticised for taking the quite untypical case of farmer Willie's scurvy, and for using it to reinforce my condemnation of the eating habits of the rural Scot. Bachelor households are known to be prone to dietary deficiencies, which may cause a very few isolated cases of florid scurvy; but the deficiencies of the McTosh's larder with its tinned meat, white bread, margarine and tinned jam is only by a slight degree worse than those of many of the households in our practice.

A few days before starting to write this chapter I visited a friend in our local cottage hospital. Supper was being served. The menu? bully beef, canned beans, white bread and jam! Maybe it is unfair to take Sunday supper as typical, but although in many hospitals there is a welcome move towards 'health foods', in others overcooked, processed foods will do nothing to promote healing.

Was Willie's scurvy the tip of an iceberg representing thousands of families suffering from what some writers have called 'sub-clinical scurvy' – that is, vitamin C deficiency not quite severe enough to cause widespread bleeding, but still likely to impair bodily defences?

Vitamin C, found in fresh fruits, berries, green leaf and root vegetables and in potato tubers, is an extraordinarily versatile substance; without it, the 'cement' holding certain cells together will loosen and break, hence the abnormal bleeding, the breakdown of wound scars and delay in healing. It is a vitamin which plays an important part in our ability to cope with bodily stress and which, as we have seen, may be protective against cancer.

As for the many items in our daily diet, experts do not agree on the minimum intake essential for health. Authorities in Britain say 30 milligrams, in the USA 60 milligrams,[3] nor is there agreement that 'sub-clinical deficiency' does exist.[4] Nobel prize-winner Linus Pauling, in his book *Cancer and Vitamin C*, argues that human beings require a daily dose not of 30 or 60 milligrams, but of between 2,300 and 12,000 milligrams.[5] A fresh lettuce, weighing 3 ounces, contains about 15 milligrams of the vitamin; so to satisfy Dr Pauling, from natural sources we would have to consume about 153 lettuces every day! Pauling supports his claim with the argument that our ape ancestors lived in lush tropical lands where an abundance of fruits and green leaf foods would make possible consumption of enormous quantities of vitamin C. He may be right, but recent research does not appear to confirm claims, based on Pauling's work, that huge daily doses of powdered vitamin C prevent the common cold or are successful in treating cancer. I doubt if we were meant to get our vitamins from a factory, and there is some evidence that taking vitamin C powder daily in heaped tablespoonfuls is not without its dangers.[6]

Again, readers are reminded of McCarrison's down-to-earth research. The peoples he studied, whose excellent health included freedom from abdominal cancer, got their vitamins from fresh fruits and vegetables, eaten in quantities easily available from the harvests of settled agriculture in any part of the temperate zone. What is so sad about the case of Willie's scurvy is that his farm was set in a south-facing, sheltered glen, where a few simple exercises in horticulture would have given him and his brother all the water-soluble vitamins they required.

The dietary regime of the Haugh farm must have resulted in multiple vitamin deficiency. Vitamin C is only one of the substances, essential for health, which is found in fruits and vegetables and which is so sorely lacking in Scotland's food. Another water-soluble vitamin, folic acid, will be discussed later, but in the next chapter I wish to give another historical example of the refusal of professional leaders to accept evidence of simple explanations for the cause of serious disease.

3. R. Passmore and M. A. Eastwood, *Human Nutrition and Dietetics* (Edinburgh, Churchill Livingstone, 1986), p. 148
4. *Ibid.*, p. 151
5. L. Pauling and E. Cameron, *Cancer and Vitamin C* (Institute of Science and Medicine, California, 1979)
6. Passmore and Eastwood, *Human Nutrition and Dietetics*, p. 150

12   Simple Causes

Night calls at certain times of the year do have their compensation. In midsummer the sun goes down behind the hills of the Faragon ridge at 9.30 p.m. and after only a few hours of half-darkness, comes up from the northeastern skyline. By 4.30 a.m. on a good day, sunlight is streaming on the valley and has a quality of mystery and magic found only at this time of year.

June 1953.   Nurse phoned at 4 a.m. Would I come to Mrs Brown? Her fourth baby had been born at the farm without difficulty, but a tear would have to be repaired. The usual agony of being hauled from sleep and bed soon gives way to a sense of wonder at the feel of summer dawn – wisps of mist by the river, and light of a peculiar radiance.

Mrs Brown and her family occupied a bothy which was part of the rectangular farm steading. The benefits of an electric supply and the convenience of sterilised instrument packs had not yet arrived in the 1950s, so I would have to sterilise my instruments by boiling for the recommended twenty minutes. Nurse and I chose the cleanest pot in the kitchen and put the instruments to boil on the Calor gas stove while we prepared the bedroom upstairs. When the instruments were ready, I poured the boiling water down the sink and, in the hope of hastening the cooling process, leaned across to an open window and held the pot in the cooler air outside. To my horror, a huge muzzle belonging to a massive cart horse was thrust to the rim of the pot. He had been lurking out of sight and was, I suppose, used to getting the odd titbit through the window; maybe from disgust at what he found in the pot, he let out a long stertorous snort.

In my mind's eye I saw the fearful cascade of equine bacteria, viruses and fungi which were thus showered on my precious tools;

there was nothing for it but to wash the lot in soap and water and start all over again. The horror of puerperal or childbed fever looms large in the teaching of obstetrics. Its cause has now been known for over a century, and the disciplines of cleanliness and asepsis are deeply implanted in the minds of nurses and medical students as they tend women in labour. The controversies which raged in the nineteenth century over measures to prevent the high mortality of childbed fever give a dramatic example of the refusal of scientists to accept the efficacy of simple measures for the prevention of serious disease, however compelling the evidence.

In 1847 a physician of Vienna, Ignaz Semmelweiss, sought by intensive study to find out why so many mothers who came to have their babies in hospital caught childbed fever and died of this dread disease.[1] He and his students spent much of their time in the post-mortem room where, in the examination of diseased organs, they hoped to find the vital clues which would lead to cure or prevention. One aspect of the disease was beyond doubt; its occurrence and mortality was far higher in the wards where students conducted the deliveries, than in the ward where only midwives were in charge. Midwives did not attend post-mortems. A friend of Semmelweis who injured himself while doing a post-mortem became ill and died after enduring feverish symptoms very similar to those suffered by women who died of childbed fever. This confirmed Semmelweiss's suspicion that the disease was contagious and was being transmitted by doctors and students. He ordered his students to wash their hands thoroughly in antiseptic solution before attending women in labour and between each case. The dramatic fall in the number of cases in the student wards following this simple measure fully confirmed the theory of contagion by some kind of infective agent (this was before Pasteur had discovered the existence of bacteria).

As in the case of scurvy and lemon juice, here was a simple way of preventing a disease 'fatal and dreadful'. Alas for human nature, the response of the Viennese doctors was exactly the same as that of Lind's eighteenth-century colleagues. They poured scorn on Semmelweiss's findings and urgent recommendations. He was brutally frank with himself and with other doctors. He realised that the soaring mortality which had followed his intensive dissecting in the post-mortem room had been caused by him and his students as

---

1. *Chambers Biographical Dictionary* (Edinburgh, Constable, 1978), p. 1157, entry on Ignaz Philip Semmelweiss

they passed infected material from corpse to ward. 'Consequently must I here make my confession that God only knows the numbers of women whom I have consigned prematurely to the grave', he wrote.[2] That was a brave thing to say, and should have commanded respect from other doctors; but they said he was talking nonsense. He responded by calling them murderers, for which he was sacked from his hospital job. In his book, *A History of Medicine*, Brian Inglis writes, in describing this episode, 'Of the countless instances of professional blindness when confronted with a reasonable hypothesis backed by convincing evidence, the opposition to Semmelweiss is the most saddening.'

The evidence collected by Cleave which demonstrates a simple cause for the serious and often fatal diseases listed above (page 60) seems to me to be no less convincing than that published in Vienna in the hope of banishing the scourge of childbed fever. The discoveries of Pasteur and the work of Lister in time vindicated Semmelweiss. I wonder how long it will be before Cleave's work receives similar recognition.

---

2. Brian Inglis, *A History of Medicine* (London, Weidenfeld and Nicolson, 1965), p. 154

13 Birth in a Tent

The night bell which rings just outside our bedroom door has a 'last trump' quality, a hideous, penetrating clang which accentuates to the full all the horror of being rudely awakened at 2 a.m. The hateful essence of the whole process is often made a thousand times worse by the impatience of the ringer who, in his anxiety, tends to forget that it takes time for you to awake, tumble out of bed, grope for dressing gown and slippers and stumble downstairs, through the surgery to the street door. And so he rings again. The second shattering ring catches you about halfway down the stairs, wakens the baby and sets off the spaniel in the kitchen on a spasm of barking; the terrier in the house across the street takes up the chorus, and you vow, as you reach the street door amid such an awful symphony, that you have had enough; on the morrow you will seek other employment.

On a December night the effects of this nocturnal torture were not alleviated by the sight of the features of Jimmy McTurk as he stood in the pool of light cast by the street lamp.

'Ma wife's nae weel.'

'What's the matter with her?'

'She's just nae weel.'

'Yes, but what's she complaining of?'

'She's just nae weel, we'll be needin' the ambulance to take her to the hose-pital.'

There seemed to be little point in prolonging the discussion. The McTurks were one of the several families of travelling folk who at that time lived in the valley in huts or tents. So far it had been very difficult to persuade them to come for antenatal care and to book a bed for delivery in the cottage hospital; from time to time, hectic calls for unexpected births in strange places ensured that rural practice was never dull. On this occasion I was unable to find out if Mrs McTurk was in labour. She had been delivered of her eighth, as far as I could remember, not very long ago, and in any case the maternity ward of the hospital was already overfull. Matron had absolutely refused to accept any further admissions.

The only possible action was to go and see what was happening. I knew that Jimmy would not ask for help if he did not really need it. In case this was a confinement, I telephoned the nurse and asked her to rendezvous with me where the path to the McTurk encampment joined the main road.

The tent stood in a clump of oak trees beside a sandpit. The December night was clear and crisp and the grass glistened white with frost as nurse and I left our cars. The tent was the usual design, made of hazel hoops stuck in the ground with tattered canvas thrown over and a hole in the middle as a chimney for the smoke from the wood fire. As we approached, Jimmy, who had preceded us on his bicycle, was shepherding his children to the shelter of the trees; the thought of them shivering there gave me doubts about the wisdom of my decision to come and see.

The stove in the middle of the tent, improvised from an old oil drum, was red-hot and flames leapt upwards from its brim. For a 'bed' on which the whole family slept there was a low recess at one end of the tent and from this dark hole Mrs McTurk's lamentations were loud. She was in labour; of that there was no doubt. As under-graduates we are taught, when diagnosing late pregnancy, how to determine by palpation which way round the baby is lying, but I doubt if our teachers ever imagined a situation where it was necessary to palpate in order to find out which way round the *mother* was lying!

However, we fixed up a torch and discovered that all was well – baby's head low in pelvis, second stage starting. The greatest hazard for the moment was the risk of a severe burn to the backside of the examiner; the tent was not very large, and while bending over to examine Mrs McTurk I was uncomfortably aware of the proximity of the central furnace.

After about thirty minutes the head duly appeared, but although contractions were strong, did not advance. Again I doubted the wisdom of staying in the tent; the prospect of a forceps delivery in this place was too awful to contemplate, maybe it had been foolish not to send for the ambulance. At this point, Mrs McTurk rose from her couch and squatted – now there were three of us squatting by the fire as if participating in some strange ritual. The change worked; a few minutes later the head crowned and nurse helped it out, face to pubis. The third stage gave no trouble, and in a short time Jimmy and his flock filed back into the tent into the warmth and, I suppose, into the family bed.

A half-moon was shining through the branches of the oak trees as nurse and I retreated thankfully to our cars. The land seemed gripped yet more firmly in the silence of midwinter, broken for a moment by a faint newborn cry from the tent.

Travelling folk and folic acid

Mrs McTurk's labour is mentioned not only as an example of birth in strange places in rural practice, but because of the high incidence of deficiency of another vitamin, which at that time seemed to be particularly common among the travelling folk of Perthshire. The vitamin in question was folic acid; lack of adequate intake causes a severe form of anaemia (megaloblastic). The only two severe cases seen in the practice so far had been in travelling-folk mothers. Discussion with the Perth Royal Infirmary obstetric unit confirmed a high incidence of this form of anaemia among tent-dwelling families in other parts of the country.

As its name suggests, folic acid is found in the foliage of green leaf vegetables; wholewheat bread is a richer source than white; other good sources are liver and kidney. Like vitamin C, folic acid is one of nature's vital substances; it plays a part in the construction of cell nuclei and so is essential for the normal growth of cells, hence the greater need for it during pregnancy; nature always gives precedence to the baby's needs, so deficiency in the mother is prone to occur during the later months of pregnancy, when, if she lacks good food, maternal vitamin stores are exhausted.[1]

At one time the relative rarity of severe megaloblastic anaemia in pregnancy seemed to indicate that deficiency of folic acid was uncommon. However, new methods of measuring evolved in the 1950s revealed that, especially among lower-income groups, even before frank anaemia became manifest, deficiency was common.[2] In the 1960s this deficiency was linked with complications of pregnancy such as premature separation of the placenta, bleeding, miscarriage and foetal deformities.[3]

One of the most tragic examples of foetal deformity is the failure of development of spinal cord and spine called spina bifida. Scotland

1. C. G. Barnes, *Medical Disorders in Obstetric Practice* (Oxford, Blackwell, 1970), p. 178
2. M. H. Hibberd and E. D. Hibberd, 'Aetiological Factors in Abruptio Placentae', *BMJ*, 5370, vol. 2 (1963), pp. 1430–36
3. *Ibid*

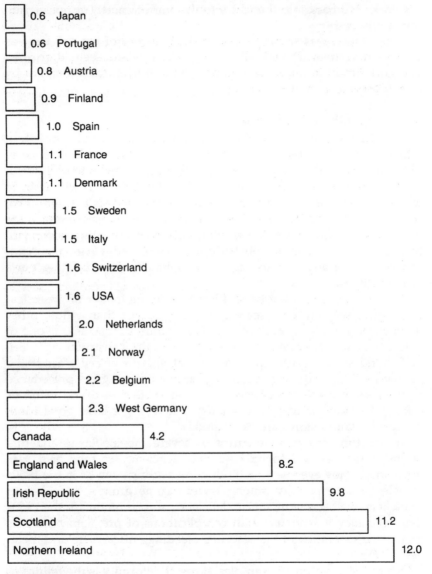

0.6 Japan

0.6 Portugal

0.8 Austria

0.9 Finland

1.0 Spain

1.1 France

1.1 Denmark

1.5 Sweden

1.5 Italy

1.6 Switzerland

1.6 USA

2.0 Netherlands

2.1 Norway

2.2 Belgium

2.3 West Germany

Canada 4.2

England and Wales 8.2

Irish Republic 9.8

Scotland 11.2

Northern Ireland 12.0

Deaths per 10,000 total births

Fig. 9: *Deaths from spina bifida in first year, 1973 (Data: WHO, 1973–76)* (*Source: Margaret and Arthur Wynn,* Prevention of Handicap and Health of Women, *London, Routledge and Kegan Paul, 1979)*

has, with Northern Ireland, the unenviable reputation of the highest incidence of spina bifida in the world (see fig. 9). As noted above (chapter 3) Margaret and Arthur Wynn have researched the occurrence of 'epidemics' of foetal (or congenital) malformations, including those of the spinal chord, during recent European history.[4] They give striking evidence which incriminates malnutrition around the time of conception as the culprit.

Multiple deficiencies

Malnutrition always brings multiple deficiencies; diets lacking foods rich in folic acid will certainly lack other vitamins and probably be deficient in minerals as well. A student of McCarrison need not concern himself or herself with details of various vitamins. I did not know about the full implication of folic deficiency when, in 1950, I composed a little diet sheet for the pregnant women coming for antenatal care, which urged them to eat wholewheat bread and at least one salad dish a day. (I reminded them that raw cabbage could be used in winter.)

The profession at large responded rather differently to the discovery of the protective role of folic acid. A pill containing iron and folic acid was advised to be taken routinely by all pregnant women, and is still being prescribed today. No cry has come from the Royal College of Obstetricians for decent bread and whole food. The prescribed folic acid will certainly prevent deficiency of that vitamin, but what about the other vitamins, minerals and fibre? For many mothers who take them, the pills will bring indigestion and constipation.

Cabbages and bulls

Over the fence from the tent in which lived Mrs McTurk's kinswoman with her folic acid deficiency anaemia, lay a field of about seven acres on which there flourished a splendid crop of winter cabbages; these were fodder for a herd of prize shorthorn bulls. Here is a picture of Scotland's nutritional disaster – plenty of folic acid for bulls, but precious little for the humans who tend them. As in the case of Willie McTosh, dying of scurvy beside a fertile field, here is a mother

---

4. Margaret Wynn and Arthur Wynn, *Prevention of Handicap and the Health of Women* (London, Routledge and Kegan Paul, 1979), p. 26

seriously ill for want of natural food growing in abundance all around her. This deprivation is not limited to the McToshes or the McTurks; they are merely extreme examples of a trend which is worldwide: the divorce of men and women from the bounty of their land.

14 Angus, Jock and their Insulin

The district nurse at Inverglen village was not given to sending unnecessary calls, so when the phone rang and her voice, vibrant with urgency, said 'Oh doctor, come quickly please, it's Angus, I must run back to him,' there was nothing for it but to go, even if the place was about eight miles away and the hour was 3 a.m. on an autumn morning.

At this hour, what dramatic scenes of nocturnal wildlife are illuminated in the headlight's beam! Here an owl, motionless on a fence post, waiting with immobile patience to pounce on a scurrying mouse; there a hedgehog ambling across the road; farther on, a hare which runs along in front of the car, unable, for some reason best known to itself, to run off to the safety of the fields; then a roe deer which, unlike the hare, at once leaps over the fence and into the trees with the ease and grace of a ballet dancer.

The cottage windows were all alight, the door was open. A narrow stairway led from the empty kitchen to two attic bedrooms from one of which came sounds, weird and strange. An astonishing scene was being enacted. Angus, a pleasant man, a bachelor and retired lorry driver, then in his late sixties, lived here with his two elderly, arthritic sisters. He always had a smile on his face and a friendly greeting, but now, strange to relate, he seemed to be having an all-in wrestling bout on his bed with the nurse. Clad in a grey flannel nightshirt, in this nocturnal struggle he appeared to be trying to stand on his head on the bed; his feet were somehow resting on the wall against which the bed was placed, and in this head-down position, while nurse desperately tried to restrain his struggles, the nightshirt had fallen down to his armpits revealing Angus in all his male nakedness. Every now and then he would utter a fearsome roar.

This awful spectacle was clearly having a shattering effect on the arthritic sisters, both now in their seventies. Like some Greek chorus, they were standing wailing by the bed; the elder, in the stress of the moment, had lapsed into her native Gaelic tongue and was crooning some kind of lament.

The reader's suspense over this unusual happening must now be ended; there was no mystery about the diagnosis of Angus's behaviour. Three weeks ago he had come complaining of excessive thirst and weight loss and had been sent to Perth Infirmary in order to have the diabetes, causing these symptoms, assessed and stabilised. News of his discharge from hospital four days ago and details of his self-administered protamine-zinc insulin treatment had not yet been received (the result of a failure of communication between hospital and GP which is, alas, all too frequent). Poor Angus was in the grip of a pretty brisk hypoglycaemic attack (low blood glucose).

Urgent action was called for. I had not yet learned the necessity of always carrying a few ampoules of dextrose solution for intravenous injection, so the sisters were instructed to hasten to the kitchen and to prepare any kind of sweetened drink. No doubt glad to be doing something and relieved to get away from the scene of torment, they obeyed with alacrity. They sped to the stairs as fast as their arthritic legs would permit, clumped down to the kitchen, and a hectic clatter of pans and dishes soon indicated that their preparations were well under way. In the meantime, in the hope of mobilising his liver glycogen reserves, I gave Angus an injection of 0.5 ml. of 1:1000 adrenalin.

The first cup soon arrived and was presented to Angus's tightly clenched dentures through which, between roars, he was hissing and blowing. Our professor of physiology, in one of his rare attempts at humour, used to illustrate the power of peristalsis or contraction in the swallowing reflex by telling an anecdote of a beer-swilling student who could drink a pint of beer standing on his head. As Angus's feet were still well above his head, I hoped that his oesophageal peristalsis was in good shape, otherwise the sugar which was urgently needed for absorption into his blood stream as glucose would not reach his stomach. But before this could be put to the test, with a sudden blow of his uppermost hand he dashed the cup from his lips and its contents all over the bedclothes and over my trousers. Undismayed, the sisters sped back to the kitchen for refill, while nurse and I continued our efforts to keep Angus horizontal.

Footsteps on the stairs heralded the approach of another cup. But it did not arrive. Instead, there was a dreadful crash, an agonised cry and the sound of falling timber, crockery and plaster. This was too much; to start the night with an intractable hypoglycaemic coma and end with a fractured neck of femur was more than flesh could bear. I rushed to the stairs to see what had happened. The wooden banister, attached to the wall by a couple of brackets, unused to this night's hectic strains had come adrift from its moorings and crashed onto the stairs. The latter were strewn with broken plaster, mingled with the contents of the second cup. By a miracle, the bearer had not fallen and already she had retreated to the kitchen for a third replacement.

By the time it arrived we had managed to get Angus's feet off the wall. Whether it was the one or two gulps he at last managed to take, or whether my adrenalin injection had had the desired effect, we will never know, but with extraordinary suddenness he sat bolt upright, gave us a beaming smile and said, 'It's yourself, doctor; man, I'm right glad to see you,' and warmly shook me by the hand.

The amiability of Angus may have been the cause of his downfall. As some hurried ward sister or nurse expounded to him the mysteries of insulin dosage, the care of syringes and the techniques of self-injection, I could see him smiling and nodding, even though he had no very clear idea what it was all about. When, on visiting him the next day, I asked him to show me on the syringe how much insulin he had been giving himself every day, he replied, 'Och, about there,' and pointed his finger vaguely halfway up the syringe. This difficulty was solved by marking the correct dose with a piece of adhesive tape. Nurse and I in conference decided that excessive dosage of insulin was a greater danger than any possible loss of sterility in the syringe. Angus's vision was already deteriorating because of the diabetic cataracts in both of his eyes. He confessed later to having difficulty in seeing the syringe markings. (Both the cataracts were later removed; he lived to the ripe age of ninety.)

The discovery of insulin and its use by injection have transformed the lives of diabetics. Will we ever find a way of delivering substitute insulin so that the amount released varies according to the level of blood sugar and thus prevents these chaotic episodes of insulin-induced coma which are such a trial to diabetics and to those who look after them? 'Chaotic episodes' similar to the nocturnal visit to Inverglen village sometimes give rise to calls to strange places.

The police-sergeant looked extremely embarrassed when I called at the police-station in answer to his message. Mr Wood, a retired accountant, church elder and respected member of his village community, was sitting in the office with a faraway look in his eyes and a rather silly grin on his face. His car had crashed through the wooden fence bordering the Kenmore road and had just been stopped by a tree from plunging into the river Tay. In this predicament Mr Wood had been verbally incoherent and inclined to laugh. This was in the days before the routine blood alcohol test, when convictions for 'drunk in charge' of a car often depended on the evidence of the doctor called to examine the suspect and pronounce on his state of intoxication. I explained to the sergeant that Mr Wood was an insulin-dependent diabetic. The blood sample which I took gave a glucose level of 40 mgm. per cent (normal level is about 80 mgm. per cent). No charge was made.

With strange thoughtlessness Mr Wood had gone out to his garden just before lunch to do some heavy gardening; the energy thus expended, plus the long-acting substitute insulin had used up his glucose which, at that time of the day, was in urgent need of replenishment by lunch. The mental confusion induced by falling blood glucose leads to actions which are quite unpredictable. Mr Wood had no recollection at all of going to his garage, getting the car out and then driving off into the blue. Unfortunately, his wife, busy in the kitchen, did not hear the car moving until it was too late. She probably would have recognised his irrational actions and given him the food required to restore normal mental function.

Diabetics seem to vary greatly in their awareness of the threat of mental confusion leading to coma, when their blood sugar begins to fall below the danger level. They are taught to carry, without fail, a sweet biscuit or sugar lump, so that at the first hint of hypoglycaemic coma they can restore blood glucose to normal; but for some, loss of mental control seems to come too swiftly to allow time for the preventive snack. Such a one was Jock the roadman, who on many occasions had to be brought round from deep coma. His attacks were not prevented by repeated referral to the consultant's diabetic clinic and by several changes of insulin regime.

As I hurried home for lunch one day, I passed Jock, sitting on a roadside dyke, his flask and sandwich box unopened beside him. Did he have a faraway look in his eye? was he teetering on the brink of coma? The feeling that my own blood sugar needed restoring after a long morning's visiting round persuaded me to believe that, with his lunch by his side, he must be about to eat; like the priest and the Levite on the road to Jericho, I weakly passed by on the other side. I had time only for a few mouthfuls before the phone rang. Geordie the woodman, phoning from a cottage not far from where Jock had been sitting, asked me to come quickly.

Geordie's squad had carried Jock's senseless body from beside the wall to a clearing where they had just felled a beech tree. They had laid him beside a huge bonfire and willingly helped to hold his arm still – he was apt to twist and turn in the restlessness which is such a distressing feature of hypoglycaemia – so that the intravenous dextrose solution could be administered with the least possible delay. The speed of Jock's return to consciousness as the solution was run into his vein deeply impressed Geordie and his men; the blazing fire gave a festive air to his recovery which, they insisted, must be celebrated with a drink all round.

These cases are dramatic examples of the well-known physiological truth that the constituents which make up body fluids, including blood, must always be kept within normal ranges. The normal range of blood glucose is between 80 and 180 mgm. per cent; secretion of insulin is the mechanism for maintaining this normality, and severe mental disturbance and possibly death result when, owing to insulin overdose, glucose level falls and cannot be restored.

The consequences are every bit as serious when in untreated diabetics blood glucose levels rise well beyond the 180 mgm. per cent level. In this event, the grossly abnormal glucose levels appear to act as a toxic agent which causes widespread tissue damage, especially in arteries, including the coronary arteries. The association of diabetes with coronary thrombosis and their cause, according to Cleave's teaching, will be discussed in the following four chapters.

15   Overconsumption

So far, in the early chapters of this book, I have attempted to highlight the sad deficiencies of the diet of the average Scottish highlander – deficiencies of vitamins, minerals, trace elements and laxative fibre. Highly processed, unfresh food may well be deficient also in essential proteins and fats and also lacking in important food factors which we know not of. I have touched on some of the evidence which links those dietary failings with the causes of constipation, varicose veins, colonic cancer, diverticular disease, difficulties in child birth and certain congenital defects.

But in the preceding chapter the encounter with diabetes brings us face to face with a disease, the main cause of which is not deficiency, but surfeit. McCarrison repeatedly pointed out that dietary deficiency and surfeit were simply different sides of the same coin. His 'poor class British diet'[1] featured tinned meat, boiled cabbage, white bread, margarine, tinned jam and plenty of refined sugar. In such a diet, the refining of carbohydrates at one stroke creates deficiency and surfeit; vitamins, minerals, proteins, fibre, etc. are removed, but the final product is excessively loaded with refined sugar and starch. Cleave has elaborated this unfortunate development and arguing from the Darwinian teaching of adaptation,[2] has used the term 'overconsumption' to describe the response of the human body to a situation, never before encountered in the long march of evolution.

Simplicity again

The concept of overconsumption is simple and yet so completely neglected in the debate on food and health that I feel compelled to enlarge on it here. Readers should turn to fig. 3 on p. 57. Let us first suppose that the ten grammes of sugar had never been refined out of

---

1. R. McCarrison, *Nutrition and Health* (Brentwood, Westbury Press, 1982), p. 29
2. T. L. Cleave, *The Saccharine Disease* (Bristol, John Wright, 1974), p. 2

its parent beetroot. When the latter is chewed and swallowed the sugar reaches the small intestine mixed with and diluted by a far greater quantity of beetroot pulp. It is then absorbed through the wall of the intestine at a relatively slow rate, a rate which is natural, because sugar does not occur on its own in nature; it occurs always as part of a plant, either cane, fruit or root. The need to chew the substance of the plant is another check on rate of sugar absorption.

Now, by industrial refining take the sugar from its plant, always remembering that without the use of slaves or machinery bulk production of refined sugar would be impossible; swallow the sugar as confectionery or sweetened drink, the rate of ingestion is about ten times the normal;[3] a surge of glucose enters the blood and puts an unnatural strain on the systems by which the body deals with it. This is what is meant by overconsumption. The chain of events is similar when refined white bread is eaten instead of wholewheat. It takes more time to chew wholewheat than white, and the removal of fibre in the bran allows the starch of the grain to be more swiftly ingested and converted into glucose. The extent of overconsumption, however, is far less when white flour is eaten than in the case of refined sugar, but overconsumption still occurs *only in the ingestion of refined carbohydrate foods*; no other foodstuffs are thus concentrated by refining. Overconsumption is of immense importance because of the major part it plays in the cause of three of the killing diseases of our time. These are obesity, diabetes and coronary thrombosis. Overconsumption is not the same thing as gluttony; it is the consequence of satisfying the appetite by eating food which has been unnaturally concentrated.

Nature's checks and balances

I can still recall the strong sense of wonder which I experienced when in 1936 I embarked as a medical student on the study of the human body. Here was perfection of structure and function, a miracle far beyond any of the artifacts made by man; bones and joints structured exactly for their function; movement by muscles, controlled by an elaborate system of nervous impulses; the whole nourished by means of blood circulating thanks to the heart's lifelong pumping, seventy beats per minute with never a rest, twenty-four hours per day and night for seventy or eighty years or beyond. The complexity of the inner workings of human organs evokes even more wonder; myriads of cells going about their business, all with a view to defending the

---

3. G. B. Harber, K. W. Heaton, and D. Murphy, 'Depletion and disruption of dietary fibre', *The Lancet*, vol. 2 (1977) pp. 679–82

tissues under our protective skin from attack by hostile agents and to maintaining a constant temperature and constant make-up of body fluids. This constancy is achieved by systems of automatic checks and balances, one example of which is the system for controlling the level of glucose in the blood.

The glucose 'thermostat'

In health, the level of blood glucose varies between 80 and 180 mgm. per 100 ml. of blood. Elaborate measures have been evolved for preventing this blood glucose level straying beyond the upper or lower limits. The hormone insulin is one of the most important agents by which the body copes with glucose; it acts like a thermostat and ensures that as soon as glucose is absorbed during a meal, it is immediately taken up by the body and either used for fuel or stored. During digestion, messages to the insulin-producing cells of the pancreas stimulate production so that enough insulin will be available; the rising curve of blood glucose is checked and within an hour or two is brought back to the resting level.

As long as sugar is eaten in its natural form, i.e. still in the parent plant, the insulin mechanism works smoothly for a lifetime. But the surge of glucose into the bloodstream when *pure, refined* sugar is swallowed puts a severe strain on the insulin-producing cells; they have not been programmed in evolutionary history to cope with such a load; desperately they try by high productivity to keep glucose levels in check. But as, year after year, the intake of refined sugar rises, those cells become exhausted and like weary workers can no longer produce; insulin levels fall with the result that blood glucose rises unchecked and goes over the upper limit of 180 mgm. per cent. In what seems like a last effort to get rid of the excess glucose the body then pours it out via the kidneys in the urine. This is Peter Cleave's explanation of the genesis of diabetes. It is not yet widely accepted, but it seems to me to fit exactly the worldwide occurrence of the commonest form of the disease – late onset diabetes, occurring in adulthood. Diabetes in infancy or childhood is not nearly so common as the late onset type, and because of the short timescale, its cause may be different. The destruction of pancreatic insulin-bearing cells by virus or other toxic agents is the most likely explanation. Before dealing with the consequences of excessive blood sugar levels, I wish briefly to touch on the other end of the blood glucose scale.

Hypoglycaemia

This is the medical term for *low* blood sugar; an example of the most dramatic manifestation of hypoglycaemia was the case of Angus, described in the preceding chapter. The restless, disturbed and sometimes violent behaviour with occasional fits is seen only as a result of insulin overdosage in the treatment of diabetes. During times of starvation, when the body is denied regular supplies of glucose from food, blood levels are kept from falling by the mobilisation of glucose from stores of glycogen in the liver, or from body fat. Glucose for muscular activity can also be drawn from muscle proteins – hence the matchstick limbs of the tragic victims of famine. These mechanisms for maintaining blood glucose levels in times of starvation are there to protect the brain and to maintain consciousness; without oxygen and without normal glucose levels, consciousness is quickly lost. The reasons for elaborate mechanisms for maintaining blood glucose levels above the lower limit of 80 mgm. per cent are thus obvious.

Sugar damage

The threat of widespread tissue damage, which in time occurs when blood glucose levels remain far above the upper limit of 180 mgm. per cent, explains the important protective function of the insulin mechanism. The commonest form of damage associated with diabetes is arteriosclerosis, the disease of the walls of the arteries which impedes the flow of blood, sometimes causing gangrene of the limbs and coronary insufficiency in the heart. Death rates from coronary thrombosis among late onset diabetics are far higher than in the general population.[4] Very small-bore arteries (arterioles) and capillaries seem to be especially susceptible to damage and malfunction in diabetes; their leaking walls cause haemorrhages and exudates which can be seen in the retina at the back of the eye through the lens of an ophthalmascope; if urine testing has been omitted, diabetes is occasionally diagnosed during routine examination of the eye.

Hyperinsulinism

We have seen how overworked insulin-producing cells situated in the pancreas, in their struggle to keep blood glucose levels within normal limits, are at first forced to produce abnormally high levels of the hormone.

Professor John Yudkin, well known for his research on sugar meta-

---

4. T. L. Cleave, *The Saccharine Disease*, p. 107

bolism, believes that much of the damage seen in diabetics and in many non-diabetics who consume sugar in quantities usual today, is due to the excessive production of insulin – hyperinsulinism.[5] Hormones, of which insulin is an example, are often compared to the instruments of a huge orchestra, all playing without discord in the miraculous symphony of life, growth and reproduction. If one instrument, insulin, is forced to play wrong notes, the whole orchestra is apt to be thrown out of harmony.

Professor Yudkin reminds us that patients with coronary thrombosis frequently have abnormal concentrations of four hormones, insulin, thyroid hormone, cortisol and oestrogen.[6] The lower rate of coronary disease among premenopausal women suggests hormonal influence. Eugene Zieglar, a Swiss paediatrician, reviewed international statistics of height and weight and concluded that the increase in body stature and the lowering of the age of puberty during the last 150 years in Western nations was constantly related to the steady rise in sugar consumption.[7] In Northern Canada Otto Schaeffer[8] recorded a marked acceleration of growth and a lowering of the age of puberty in Inuit (Eskimos) living in trading townships where, in contrast to their traditional diet, they ate less food from animal sources and quadrupled their consumption of sugar.

These studies from Europe and from Canada certainly link changes in growth and abnormal levels of sex hormones with the eating of sugar in quantities prevailing in industrial nations. Whether or not damage to arteries and to other tissues (nerves, kidneys, eyes) found so frequently in diabetics is due primarily to high blood glucose levels, or to disturbance of hormone 'harmony', we do not know; but to emphasise the difficulties facing anyone attempting to retain an open mind on these details of biochemistry, I feel bound to mention new research suggesting yet another explanation of why some diabetics and even non-diabetics should suffer premature degeneration of various bodily systems.

Abnormal 'glycation'

Since the 1960s it has been known that glucose molecules attach them-

5. J. Yudkin, *Pure White and Deadly* (London, Penguin Books, 1988), p. 5
6. J. Yudkin, 'Sucrose, coronary heart disease, diabetes and obesity: Do hormones provide a link?', *American Heart Journal*, 115, no. 2 (1988), pp. 493–8
7. E. Zieglar, 'Secular changes in the stature of adults and the secular trend of modern sugar consumption, *Zeitschrift für Kinderheilkunde*, 99 (1967), p. 146
8 O. Schaeffer, 'Pre and post natal growth acceleration and increased sugar consumption in Canadian Eskimos', *Journal of the Canadian Medical Association*, 103 (1977), p. 1055

selves to certain protein molecules as part of the normal work of cells in the bodies of animals and man; the process is called 'glycosylation' or 'glycation' of protein. But in the last five years scientists have discovered that in diabetics and even in non-diabetics with abnormally high blood glucose levels, glucose tends to latch on to protein molecules in an uncontrolled fashion which may have serious consequences. As always in biochemistry, details of glycation are very complicated. They were reviewed recently by Anna Furth,[9] who suggested that when glycation is uncontrolled because of persisting high blood glucose levels, abnormal proteins emerge which may lead to defective tissue structures and to such common disorders as osteoporosis (fragile bones in the elderly), arteriosclerosis and cataract. Dr Furth writes:

> So glycation may have debilitating effects on many different areas of body function – fat and cholesterol metabolism, blood clotting, intracellular and extracellular support . . . Kidney, circulatory and neurological problems are among the complications of diabetes, with athereosclerosis often being the major cause of death. Cataracts are common. Many of these problems involve glycation of three long-lived proteins – collagen, myelin or crystallin.

(Collagen is an important constituent of the joints, ligaments and associated supporting structures; myelin of the nerves; crystallin of the lens of the eye.)

It is too early to know the full significance of this new work. But we need not get lost in the biochemical trees; what matters is the shape of the wood, which fully confirms Cleave's insistence on the far-reaching effects of overconsumption and his belief that diabetes and coronary thrombosis occur simply because the human body was not evolved to withstand unnaturally high blood glucose levels, which follow repeated ingestion of large quantities of refined sugar.

Incubation period

The worldwide spread of diabetes which follows the change from traditional, natural foods to refined carbohydrates, and the increase in incidence of the disease in the UK during this century, follow a similar pattern. Cleave has compared this pattern to the lighting of a fuse when the consumption of refined sugar approaches 90 lb. per

---

9. Anna Furth, 'Sweet Peril for Proteins', *New Scientist*, 1602, vol. 117 (1988), pp. 58–62

head of population per annum.[10] Between the lighting of the fuse and the 'explosion' of the disease there is a pause or incubation period which varies in length according to the disease. For diabetes the length is about twenty years, for coronary thrombosis, thirty years, for diverticular disease, forty years (see fig. 12 in chapter 18, p. 137).

Fig. 11 on p. 133, illustrating the steep rise in sugar consumption in the UK since the beginning of the nineteenth century, puts the time of the lighting of the 90-lb.-per-head fuse in the closing decade of that century; hence the beginnings of the diabetes and coronary thrombosis 'epidemic' in the 1920s and 1930s. Similar examples of the incubation periods have been observed in other countries.

Diabetic history

Unfortunately, no reliable diagnostic records were kept in the Aberfeldy practice to confirm with precision the impression among the doctors of a great increase in the numbers of diabetics during the decades following World War II. There was, at any rate, no doubt at the Aberfeldy chemist that the numbers of prescriptions for insulin had increased enormously during that period. Until the eighteenth century, the disease seems to have been very rare.[11] Since the discovery of insulin in the 1920s in Canada by Banting and Best and the introduction of treatment based on the control of blood sugar by insulin injections, the outlook for diabetics had been transformed and death rates are maybe no longer an accurate reflection of the incidence in any population enjoying the benefits of modern treatment; the latter is now greatly improved by the use of new oral medicaments, but records suggest that from the middle of the nineteenth century death rates from diabetes rapidly increased until 1950.[12]

In chapter 18, while discussing coronary thrombosis, I shall refer to nature's experiments worldwide, which repeatedly have shown the arrival of coronary disease of the heart as populations abandon their traditional diets and take to modern foods. Exactly the same thing happens in the case of diabetes; the Canadian Inuit, whose stature and sexual development were noted above, now suffer from diabetes as frequently as other advanced populations.[13] Their plight is similar to that of Icelanders whose traditional diet consisted of 80–85 per cent proteins and fats; these animal foods are now reduced to some 45 per

10. T. L. Cleave, *The Saccharine Disease*, p. 107
11. H. C. Trowell and D. P. Burkitt, *Western Diseases: Their Emergence and Prevention* (London, Edward Arnold, 1981), p. 24
12. T. L. Cleave, *The Saccharine Disease*, p. 82
13. *Ibid.*, p. 90

cent and their place has been taken by refined carbohydrates featuring a high intake of sugar of over 100 lb per head per annum; diabetes is now common in Iceland, where even in 1938 it was still very rare.[14] Some textbooks still include the supposed stress of the urban life in modern societies as the explanation for the appearance of diabetes among 'primitive' peoples as they change from traditional to western life styles. Before continuing the theme of overconsumption as the cause of coronary thrombosis I shall attempt in the next chapter to explain why I believe stress plays a minor role in the cause of modern diseases.

---

14. *Ibid.*, p. 92

16   Duodenal Ulcer, Stress and Food-Combining

The blood, which Mrs Moss had so suddenly and so copiously vomited, covered everything around her – nightdress, bedclothes, carpet and furniture; she must, I thought, have lost a couple of pints. Now she lay back in bed, her deathly pallor and anxious expression typical signs of surgical shock which follows copious blood loss.

There are few more daunting emergencies in general practice than massive gastrointestinal bleeding, without blood transfusion the outcome may be fatal and often, in rural practice, many miles separate the patient from the nearest blood bank. To keep Mrs Moss's circulation from failing I would have to set up an intravenous drip and in all haste go with her to Perth Royal Infirmary in the ambulance; bleeding such as this usually stops of its own accord, but has to be closely monitored in a hospital where fresh blood is at hand. Luckily, her husband and son were there to help carry her and the drip bottle with its tubing and the cannula strapped to her arm down the narrow stairs of the cottage and into the ambulance.

The thirty-mile journey seemed an eternity; in a swaying vehicle it is not easy to keep a regular and accurate check on pulse and blood pressure, nor to be sure that the cannula may not have slipped out of the vein. On this occasion all was well. The duty doctor at Perth had been warned of our coming and the drip set was still in place to take the blood bottles which had been reserved for us.

Mrs Moss had for long suffered from acid-type dyspepsia; the duodenal ulcer causing her symptoms had on this evening eroded into an artery, which had poured blood into her stomach. She was a plump, apparently contented lady, wife of the forester and mother of a large family. They all seemed to live busy, contented lives in this cottage up by the burn, surrounded by dogs, hens, ducks and other assorted livestock. It would be difficult to find anyone less like the high-powered, commuting executive, supposed to be the typical ulcer sufferer.

Ulcer history

As mentioned in earlier chapters, duodenal ulcer is one of a group of diseases which, from being extremely rare until the end of the last century, is now a common cause of distress and disability,[1] a history which it shares with diabetes, coronary thrombosis and appendicitis. It cannot too often be stressed that these are truly new diseases of our time: this simple fact is often forgotten by those who search for cause and thus for prevention.

These diseases are sometimes known as 'diseases of civilization' because of their rarity among certain isolated 'primitive' peoples. We have seen how, during his nine years as medical officer to the Hunzas, isolated in their Himalayan valley, McCarrison encountered not one single case of duodenal ulcer. He noted that, apart from sensations of hunger, these cheerful people seemed unaware of their digestive tracts. They suffered from none of the distressing symptoms of indigestion ('colonic lamentations' in McCarrison's words) which, in the West, send patients in their droves to doctors' surgeries.[2]

Ulcer patterns

McCarrison contrasted the abdominal health of these northern Indian tribes with the high incidence of ulcers of the stomach and duodenum among the polished rice eaters of Madras – the 'ulcer belt' of the Indian sub-continent. He became convinced that the excellent food of the Hunzas and the Sikhs, wholewheat chapattis, dairy produce and abundance of fruits and vegetables, protected them from abdominal disasters. His conviction seemed to be strengthened by laboratory rat-feeding experiments in which colonies of rats fed on the polished rice regime were found to suffer, as did humans, from a high incidence of stomach ulcers.[3] Since writing this I have been informed by Dr Reginald Passmore, joint author of *Human Nutrition and Dietetics*, that the stomach of the rat differs so much from the human stomach that comparisons are not valid; but even if, in this instance, McCarrison's

---

1. C. F. W. Illingworth, *Peptic Ulcer* (Edinburgh, E. & S. Livingstone, 1953)
2. R. McCarrison, 'Faulty food in relation to gastrointestinal disorder' *Journal of the American Medical Association*, 18, vol. 1 (1992), pp. 1–9
3. R. McCarrison, *Nutrition and Health* (Brentwood, Westbury Press, 1982)

laboratory evidence must be dismissed, there is no disagreement about the pattern of ulcer prevalance in India.

Cleave again

McCarrison did not know why a dietary regime depending heavily on polished rice should cause peptic ulcer; Cleave's research gives us a convincing explanation. In the polishing of rice, as in the milling of wheat, much of the protein fraction of the cereal is lost in the discarded bran; in the case of sugar, the loss of protein through refining is total. Protein buffers the hydrochloric acid poured out by the stomach during digestion, thus protein-stripped foods – polished rice, white flour and above all sugar – lose their buffering action, allowing abnormally high levels of acid to build up in the stomach and erode the wall of stomach or duodenum. This process is particularly active in those who habitually take between-meal snacks of sugary foods.[4]

My belief that Cleave's theory is correct and that it points to a simple means of preventing an incalculable amount of human pain, bleeding, incapacity and expense has been strengthened by observing the healing wrought by simple dietary change. Sufferers from heart-burn and acid-type dyspepsia, often young men who take with them to their work packed lunches consisting of white bread sandwiches, cakes and sweet biscuits all washed down with sweetened tea, showed dramatic improvement if they and their wives could be persuaded to substitute wholewheat bread for white and eat fresh fruit instead of sweetened foods.

All in the mind?

The theory that peptic ulcer is caused simply by faulty food collides head on with the widespread belief that the cause is all in the mind and that ulcers are the result of the stress of modern living; for a while, that is what I believed. When, after demobilisation from service in the RAMC, I began preparing myself for civilian general practice, I became greatly interested in theories of 'psychosomatic medicine' which saw the cause of most human ailments in suppressed and therefore unconscious mental conflict. In the 1930s Freud's teaching had spread with a fervour which was not always tempered by com-monsense or a sense of humour. Psychoanalysts explained modern diseases in terms of the dynamics of infantile sexuality; warring impulses in the unconscious part of the human mind caused not

---

4. T. L. Cleave, *Peptic Ulcer* (Bristol, John Wright, 1962)

only broken human relationships, but also serious organic disease. According to these theories, Mrs Moss's ulcer must have been caused by 'an unconscious conflict between her wish to be independent and a wish to return to the maternal breast'.[5]

At that time these psychosomatic theories, although weird, seemed to me to be intriguing and important. Possibly the emotional stresses of military service which I had so recently observed in others and experienced myself added impetus to my studies. I eagerly read the works of Freud and authors of psychosomatic literature and for a while was convinced that the cause of peptic ulcer, heart disease and possibly diabetes were all expressions of inner mental conflict. But as the failure of psychoanalysis as a treatment for organic disease became apparent, the simpler concept of stress gained ground.[6]

Modern stress

The stress theory, emphasising the ill effects of stifling physical responses to emotion, finds an echo in Freud's theories of repression and in Rousseau's 'noble savage', who, left to himself in uncivilised innocence, is free from all the ills of advanced nations. If the supposed harmful effect of suppressing impulses of aggression were real, there would have been a dramatic fall in the incidence of 'stress' diseases in Britain during the last thirty years, a time when the restraints of civilisation have been thrown to the winds, when violence of word and deed are commonplace; could anything be farther from the behaviour of our boorish young of today than the advice of Polonius: 'Give thy thoughts no tongue, nor any unproportioned thought his act'.

During this century the growing influence in academic circles of theories which scorn all thought of human restraint and which reject the disciplines of religion and custom have had far-reaching consequences; they have brought forth the permissive society, chaos in our schools, a sad lowering of educational standards, increasing crime and violence and near destruction of the family as the biological unit of society.

When the cause of a new disease or group of diseases is not clear, doctors and their patients tend to blame emotional or stress factors. By 1910 acute appendicitis, a disease unknown until the closing decades of the nineteenth century, had become common enough to be the

---

5. F. G. Alexander and T. M. French, *Studies in Psychosomatic Medicine* (New York, Ronald Press, 1948)
6. H. Selye, *The Stresses of Life* (London, Longmans Green, 1957)

subject of prolonged comment in the correspondence columns of the *British Medical Journal*.[7] The following new inventions were put forward as the cause of this new disease: (a) the increasing use of the telephone, (b) the increasing use of the photographic camera, (c) riding in tram cars and (d) rushing off to work on bicycles!

Here is an interesting example from Africa of this same tendency. From the medical history of that continent it seemed clear in the 1930s that diabetes did not occur among the native peoples, living in traditional surroundings. In the Nairobi African Hospital, where every patient admitted had routine urine testing for sugar, during the three years 1930–33 the late Dr Hugh Trowell did not encounter a single case of diabetes in an African.[8] But in 1933 a case did occur, and the hospital staff met to examine this strange phenomenon.

The patient was a fat African nursemaid living in the household of her British employer. Here, those doctors decided, was a disease of civilisation brought about by the impact of the stress of western culture on an African woman conditioned to a relaxed tribal way of life. The choice of the impact of western culture and restraint, rather than of western food, demonstrates how fashion is apt to sway conclusions relating to the cause of new diseases.

The impact of reality

As my work continued year by year among the families living in this Highland strath, pyschosomatic or stress theories seemed less and less convincing as the cause of modern diseases. Freud's writings may well illuminate the complexities of human relationships and give new insights into the working of the human psyche, but, as noted above, psychoanalysis has been of no help at all either in elucidating the cause or in successfully treating diseases of civilisation; and how can the appearance of duodenal ulcer during this century be explained by a conflict between an infantile wish to remain at the maternal breast and a wish to be independent? Such conflicts, if they exist, must have been with us throughout human history; all the evidence points to duodenal ulcer as a new disease.

As for the stress of modern living by which we usually mean urban-type stress, the din and rush of the city, traffic jams or the strain of the factory, if these were important factors in causing modern diseases, peptic ulcers would be extremely rare in the Aberfeldy practice. 'No hurry, north of Dunkeld'; is a jocular saying to describe the slow

---

7. C. Mercier, letter in *BMJ*, vol. 2 (1910), p. 2003

8. H. C. Trowell and D. B. Burkitt, *Western Diseases* (London, Edward Arnold, 1981), p. 24

tempo of life in this part of the Highlands; but the so-called 'stress diseases' appear to be no less common here than in our cities. High blood pressure, ulcers, coronary heart disease and other ailments are by no means uncommon among our rural communities. Stress may often trigger a heart attack or an episode of indigestion, but I am convinced that the underlying cause is dietary.

I wish to make clear that my rejection of stress or psychological factors as the cause of twentieth-century organic diseases does not imply that I dismiss emotional disturbance as a cause of ill-health. Elsewhere I have tried to stress the immense importance of mental turmoil as a frequent cause of dramatic human reactions, such as fainting, vomiting, diarrhoea and a multitude of aches and pains for which sufferers seek their doctor's help.[9 and 10] Estimates vary on the proportion of cases in general practice which are expressions of psychological or emotional trouble; about one third used to be the accepted figure. These are cases where no organic (or structural) change in the organs of the patient can be discovered to account for his or her distress. But in all cases, whether or not organic disease is present, the wise doctor will try and understand his or her patient's emotional state of mind and if possible allay fears and loneliness. This approach can have unexpected rewards, as the following case illustrates.

The angry colonel

The retired colonel was a difficult man, a widower, who tended to fall out with friends and relations; he had a poor opinion of doctors, who could do nothing for his migraine; blinding headaches and vague feelings of indigestion forced him to lie for hours in his darkened bedroom, where he frequently injected himself with shots of ergotamine tartrate (the standard treatment, then, for control of migraine headache). Extensive investigation had found no brain tumour or other organic cause for his misery.

He came through to the sitting room when I arrived and was loud in his complaints of his own discomfort and of the uselessness of the medical profession. I began to feel pretty miserable myself and found it hard to know how to reply to this tale of woe. In a pause in the conversation, I glanced uncomfortably round the room and, for want of anything else to say, commented 'What a very beautiful chair that

9. W. W. Yellowlees, 'All the world's a stage', *Journal of the Royal College of General Practitioners*, 17, supplement 3 (1972), pp. 30–35
10. W. W. Yellowlees, 'Stress and Disease', *Update*, 12, vol. 4 (1972), pp. 1443–50

is,' and pointed to the piece in question. This innocent remark turned out to be a bull's-eye hit. 'I'm glad you like it,' he said, 'I made it.' I expressed surprised admiration for his skill.

Suddenly the tone of our consultation was transformed; with obvious pride he showed me other pieces of his handiwork. Forgotten in a flash, it seemed, was his litany of woe and calamity. He invited me to see his workshop where he enthused on the art of copying Chippendale. I had inadvertently pierced the armour of his resentment and isolation and had become an ally rather than an enemy. 'Now doctor,' he said, as I prepared to go, 'surely there is something you can give me to relieve these headaches.' Sensing that I should strike while the iron was hot, I replied yes, I was sure that his symptoms could be relieved. I advised him to stop injecting himself, to take bran daily for the relief of the constipation which was probably the cause of his abdominal discomfort and to take a new vitamin B preparation which I would prescribe.

When I returned a week later, he was a new man; injections were no longer needed, his headaches infinitely better; he was up and about all day and was sure that the marvellous vitamin 'tonic' had done the trick. In the following years he must have consumed well over a gallon of the stuff in teaspoon doses; his migraine, although not entirely cured, ceased to trouble him seriously.

I have recounted this case to illustrate the deliberate use of a placebo to help a personality who would not, in my opinion, be amenable to explanations of how his troubles were due to emotional factors. I had prescribed myself and used the 'tonic' as a token; we continued on the best of terms, though I very much doubt if the vitamins or the bran had any significant effect on his symptoms.

Food combining

I cannot leave the subject of peptic ulcer without referring to a book by Doris Grant and Jean Joice published in 1984, *Food Combining for Health*.[11] The message of this book is that in some cases the dietary improvements mentioned above in the treatment of ulcer-type indigestion may not always be successful. 'Food combining' is based on the Hay system of eating as taught by an American doctor, the late William Howard Hay. In broad outline, the theory of the system is that protein foods, such as meat, fish, poultry and game, should not be eaten at the same meal with starchy, sugary foods. Otherwise its advice on the

---

11. Doris Grant, *Food Combining for Health* (London, Thorsons Publishing Group, 1984)

quality of food, especially the value of wholewheat bread, dairy produce, fresh fruits, vegetables and salads, is in exact accord with McCarrison's teaching.

Dr Hay's account of human digestion would not be accepted by
modern physiologists; our knowledge of digestive processes, however,
is by no means complete. Mrs Grant suffered as a young woman
from chronic joint pains and indigestion; in despair at the failure of
conventional treatment she tried the Hay system, found instant relief
and has remained a lifelong adherent of this way of eating. A staunch
campaigner for wholewheat bread and for natural, health-giving food,
she is well known as an author; her books, *Your Daily Bread, Housewives
Beware, Your Daily Food*,[12] did much to educate housewives on the
importance of sound nutrition. Mrs Grant is certainly a good advertise-
ment for her beliefs; now aged eighty-eight, her interests, enthusiasms
and activities seem undimmed by age.

In a foreword to *Food Combining for Health*, the actor Sir John Mills
gives a vivid account of his invalidism as a result of a large duodenal
ulcer which hospital treatment, with its rice puddings, mashed
potatoes and such foods, failed to relieve. Within six weeks of embarking on the Hay diet, he was able to start working on a film; his ulcer
has not recurred.

Success of a system

Since publication of *Food Combining for Health*, a steady stream of
letters has flowed to the authors from grateful readers; many were
victims of chronic indigestion and of peptic ulcer. Another group of
sufferers who have found dramatic relief are those in the grip
of manifestations of food intolerance or allergy – migraine, skin rashes,
urticaria or joint pains. The book soon became a best seller; it has now
achieved thirty-seven impressions and the sale of over half a million
copies; it has been translated for Portuguese, Spanish, Greek, Israeli,
Dutch, Serbo-Croat and Finnish readers. An American edition has
been an equal success. Having had the opportunity of interviewing
several people who experienced dramatic relief of symptoms by using
the Hay system, I am sure that its success is not due to auto-suggestion
and that however much its theory may be questioned, in practice, for
a substantial number of people the system works, though not by any
means for all. Some patients will not benefit from food combining
and, as the book advises, many people get on perfectly well without

---

12. Doris Grant, *Your Daily Food* (London, Faber, 1973)

it. But if I suffered from indigestion or any other symptoms of food intolerance, the Hay system would be my first choice of treatment; it costs nothing and cannot possibly harm.

Orthodox disbelief

In expressing their gratitude to Mrs Grant, correspondents often complain of the scepticism of their doctors when the latter are told of the success of the Hay system. GPs repeatedly encounter episodes of dramatic improvements in patients like the angry colonel who are made better by suggestion, tactful handling and a little understanding of the needs of the human psyche. Orthodox doctors tend to attribute tales of miracles merely to the power of suggestion and point to the many 'quacks' thriving on the gullibility of people from all walks of life, who are attracted by bizarre methods and dramatic cures. In any case, they would argue, we now have such effective drug antagonists of hydrochloric acid which bring instant relief to ulcer sufferers, why bother with strange diets?

It is unfortunate that *Food Combining for Health* has evidently been dismissed in this way by doctors and dieticians. Case histories of success of the Hay system are too numerous and to constant to be due to suggestion or to chance. It would be comparatively easy to assess its effectiveness, with all the rigours of scientific discipline, in some large hospital department of gastroenterology; there, hundreds of cases of, say, duodenal ulcer could be invited to participate in a trial of the Hay method. How sad that this has not been done; here is a golden opportunity to do worthwhile research at very little expense; if the Hay system was shown to meet the claims of its founder, relief of suffering would be widespread without the use of acid-suppressing drugs.

Possibly official investigation has not been contemplated because highly trained scientists cannot bring themselves to believe that a housewife (Mrs Grant) could possibly teach them anything, even though she is reviving the work of a qualified doctor. However much those scientists might question Dr Hay's theories of human digestion, if his system works, that is what matters. In spite of dazzling advances in understanding of physiology there remain vast areas of ignorance; this is true of digestive processes and of the cause or causes of food intolerance. There is so much we do not understand.

17   Rheumatism, Homeopathy: Physician Heal Thyself

The scorn of orthodox doctors for 'Food Combining' as a treatment for rheumatic complaints brings us to a brief discussion of rheumatic diseases. They are among the top three causes of disability in the insured population of the UK. They include well-defined diseases such as rheumatoid arthritis and osteoarthritis. To lay people, the word rheumatism means the aches, pain and stiffness of limbs, back, joints and muscles from which few of us do not suffer at some time in our lives. Rheumatic complaints have one thing in common – their cause is mostly unknown and their prevention has so far eluded us; a journey through the wilderness of medical controversy would be incomplete without mention of these common maladies.

McCarrison observed that rheumatic diseases were far more prevalent among certain poorly fed populations in the south of India than in the better fed people of the Punjab.[1] This contrast, and the distressing frequency of rheumatic complaints in Britain today, could be explained by the following three dietary factors:

1. Deficiency of vitamins, minerals, essential proteins and fats, trace elements and other necessary ingredients in food, degraded by industrial refining/processing. Such deficiency can lead to inadequate repair to cartilage, ligaments and other joint tissues, which are subject to the incessant wear and tear of weight-bearing and movement. McCarrison found that vitamin C and the B complex vitamins played a part in the normal nourishment of joints.

2. Degeneration of bones and joints as a result of abnormal glycation of protein (see chapter 15 above).

3. Severe allergies are often accompanied by joint pains and swell-

---

1. R. McCarrison, *Nutrition and Health* (Brentwood, Westbury Press, 1982), p. 51

ing. Methods are now available for identifying the food or other toxic agent which may cause such reactions.[2] We are, however, all different; one man's meat is another's poison and each case must be separately assessed. The offending food may be wheat, milk or a particular fruit. In cases of straightforward allergy the removal of the offending food brings instant relief, but in many cases no such clear-cut mechanisms can be discovered.

Vague symptoms of indigestion often accompany joint pains associated with food intolerance. If I suffered from any form of rheumatism with or without indigestion, my first search for relief would be to follow the Food Combining programme mentioned in Chapter 16.

When I first wrote that paragraph I implied that mercifully no such search for relief had for me been necessary. I had vowed, in a work on nutrition and health, not to mention my own state of health for two reasons. The first is the danger of being a bore and of being seen as an exhibitionist. The second is that my state of health could have little relevance to the arguments put forward in this book in favour of simple dietary reform. Not until I was in my thirties did I learn about McCarrison's research and begin to put his teaching into practice. Although my dear mother was a superb cook, white bread and sugar were part of our daily fare at home; and I shudder when I remember the ghastly food that I have consumed at school, university, hospital residences or in the army.

Modern research[3] has demonstrated the vital importance of sound nutrition from our very earliest years if we are to lay a strong foundation for adult health. The 'earliest years' go back to the time of conception. By middle age irreparable damage may have been done, but I liked to believe that my wife and I owed our freedom from gross manifestations of degeneration to the attempts in our household, thanks to her skill and forbearance in the kitchen, to adhere to the teaching of McCarrison and Cleave.

As I approach my seventh-fifth birthday it was perhaps unwise of me inwardly to congratulate myself on having so far escaped need for medical aid.

In the week before my birthday I was suddenly smitten by an uncommon affliction of the elderly called 'temporal arteritis', a strange inflammation of the arteries of the scalp; the headache, the pain in the

2. Richard MacKarness 'Not in the Mind' (London, Pan Books Ltd, 1976)
3. M. Wynn and A. Wynn, *Prevention of Handicap and the Health of Women* (London, Routledge and Kegan Paul, 1979)

jaw muscles when eating and episodes of blurred vision are extremely unpleasant. I hurried to my doctor and got instant relief from the fairly large dose of steroid which he prescribed. The thing is said to be self-limiting, that is, it goes away in time.

I have broken my vow not to bore readers with details of personal health because temporal arteritis belongs to a group of diseases related to some forms of rheumatism. They are sometimes called the 'auto-immune' diseases; they occur when something happens in our immune mechanism which induces us to make antibodies against our own tissues; our defending cells, instead of attacking a foreign invader, attack normal friendly tissues, in this case certain arteries of the head and scalp. Sometimes auto-immune antibodies can be detected by laboratory blood tests as in rheumatoid arthritis; in others, no diagnostic tests are so far available. Temporal arteritis is grouped as a rheumatic disease with a similar auto-immune condition of the elderly called polymyalgia rheumatica.

Why should human immune systems go wrong in this way? No one seems to know. Standard textbooks are of no help; some use the word 'idiopathic' a code word in medical jargon for 'we have no idea of the cause'. Textbooks seem reluctant even to discuss possible causes. Those suffering from this kind of condition have the impression that orthodox medicine is not particularly interested in a cause, only in classifying and in elaborating treatment.

Diseases of unknown cause give fertile ground for speculation, especially among practitioners of alternative medicine. A chance meeting with a former GP who had given up his NHS practice in order to take up homeopathy gave me a chance to learn the homeopath's belief in the true cause of many illnesses, which orthodox medicine does not understand; this takes us into deep water, or perhaps I should say dense wilderness.

To some qualified doctors homeopathy may seem ridiculous; but until a doctor has studied and practised it, he or she is in no position to write off this branch of alternative medicine. The homeopath dwells in realms different from the world as we experience it with our earthly senses. He (or she) sees chronic illness as an imbalance in vital energies which cannot be detected by conventional methods; intuition of the 'extra-sensory perception' of the individual practitioner must be brought to bear. The imbalances or inhibitions of energy (termed 'miasms' in homeopathic language) which lead to chronic ill-health may originate in childhood illness or even in ancestral diseases of which tuberculosis and syphilis are important.[4] Homeopathic remedies, 'potentiated' by exphyme dilution in accordance with the method discovered by the founder of homeopathy, Samuel C. F. Hahnemann (1755–1843), are given to correct the energy imbalance and so to restore health. The apparent success of this treatment when conventional methods have nothing to offer or have failed has ensured the survival and growth of homeopathic medicine. Courses at Glasgow's Homeopathic Hospital for NHS doctors are over subscribed.

The weakness of a system of medicine which depends on the intuition or extra-sensory perception of the practitioner is obvious; an outside observer has no means of checking diagnostic methods or findings. Nonetheless, I have no wish to dispute the existence of energy fields which we cannot detect with ordinary senses, or doubt that some doctors may by intuition be able to tap this source of energy for the cure of illness. Similar arguments apply to the teachings of Rudolf Steiner in agriculture and education. Steiner's methods seem to have been derived from his unique powers of intuition; that has not prevented his teaching from now being accepted in many farms, gardens, schools and in village communities for the mentally handicapped.

But in seeking prevention rather than cure we do not need to enter the unseen world of vital energies. We know enough with our earthly senses to conclude that dietary faults are the main cause of the diseases mentioned in this book and to predict that until those dietary faults are corrected improvement in national health will not occur.

The appearance and increase during this century of chronic diseases of industrial nations – coronary thrombosis, duodenal ulcer and diabetes, for instance – cannot be explained by acquired or inherited 'miasms'; surely, if ancestral tuberculosis leads to degenerative disease in later generations, the dramatic decline in the incidence of tuberculosis in the last fifty years would have been reflected in a decrease in the occurrence of coronary thrombosis and other such diseases, rather than the increase which has taken place.

The homeopath is maybe expressing in his own language the fact that infection in childhood can have serious long-term effects. For instance, infections of the throat by a particular bacterium, the haemolytic streptococcus, sometimes the cause of acute rheumatic fever, can result in valvular disease of the heart in later years or in acute kidney disease (nephritis). One school of thought sees childhood viral disease

---

4. J. H. Reyner, *Psionic Medicine* (London, Routledge and Kegan Paul, 1974)

as the cause of multiple sclerosis in adults. If this mechanism holds for temporal arteritis, the severe haemolytic streptococcal throat infection which I suffered as a student (from which it took months to recover), might satisfy a search for cause.

Whether it does so or not, the overall importance of nutrition as the basis of health remains unshaken. The prescription of McCarrison and Cleave for health-giving diet will prevent the occurrence or lessen the severity and complications of bacterial or viral infections. My struggle with the haemolytic streptococcus might have been much less severe had I not been subsisting on a diet high in refined starch and sugar. Throughout the world, malnourished children suffer far more from the complications of measles than the better fed. Rheumatic fever and its complications are predominantly diseases of lower-income groups.

Indigestion and the possibility of peptic ulcer are among the daunting list of side effects of steroids. I certainly experienced the most violent gripping abdominal pains within a few days of embarking on a steroid course. Strict adherence to food combining seems to have prevented any recurrence of these distressing symptoms.

18 A ken fine it's his appendix

A traveller, setting out on foot or on horseback, from Scotland's western shores at Oban or Inveraray can cross the Highlands from west to east without having to climb a single mountain ridge; such a traveller, using the cleft formed by Loch Awe, Glen Lochy, Strath Fillan, Glen Dochart, Loch Tay and finally the broad strath of the river Tay, is following a track through Scotland first used by Neolithic settlers who came in their primitive boats from Spain, Brittany or Ireland. Later Bronze Age settlers, arriving probably from Germany and the Low countries, used the same route to penetrate the Highlands from east to west.

The numerous burial mounds and standing stones raised by these prehistoric people are evidence of widespread human settlement in those far-off days; this is especially true of the central part of the cleft formed by the valley of the upper Tay in which stands the small burgh of Aberfeldy. Here on the broad valley floor, in spite of two centuries of intensive agriculture, burial mounds and impressive groups of standing stones remain; steep slopes rise from the flat cultivated fields to moorland and mountain top; the moors give wide catchment areas for the many swift-flowing burns which cascade down narrow glens to join the main river.

During the eighteenth and nineteenth centuries, water mills, usually built where the burns met the low ground, became the focus of small villages whose families worked in the new industries of milling, weaving or timber sawing; now, of course, the mill-wheels are broken and crumbled, the storehouses in ruins.

I used to think it was silly sentiment to wish that the mills were still working as centres of rural activity, but recent revelations of the consequences of depending wholly on fossil fuel or on nuclear energy are surely strong arguments in favour of reviving these simple sources of energy, unpolluting and permanent (as long as man-made climatic changes do not dry up the burns!). Such a revival has already been accomplished in Aberfeldy, where the eighteenth-century water mill, kept going during this century by the grain and food business of McKerchar and McNaughton, has now been completely renovated by Mr Tom Rodger of Cupar in Fife, and is presently milling organically grown oats.

Diagnostic triumph

To return to my case notes; the burn which flowed through the little village of Milton with its disused mill was probably the source of the trouble in the case to be recounted. Five-year-old Morag had been unwell for several days, complaining of vague symptoms of abdominal discomfort and of generally feeling tired and sick. I asked the district nurse to chart her temperature; after some three days the chart showed an alarmingly sinister pattern which I probably would not have recognised had I not the good fortune (if that is the right word) to have witnessed in 1945, in the aftermath of war, a minor outbreak of typhoid fever in north Germany.

But no case of typhoid had occurred in the practice for years; surely I was jumping to wrong conclusions. Think too of the panic a case of typhoid would provoke in the office of the then Medical Officer of Health. There was no doubt, however, when I visited her again, about the presence of the typical 'rose spot' rash on her tummy, while the white cell blood count which I had done (in those days we had to do them ourselves) was typical of typhoid.

I heard later that the staff of the distant Isolation Hospital had been duly impressed when their bacteriological tests confirmed that the GP diagnosis had been correct. Morag made a complete recovery; I had not known that in those days the outside privies at the upper end of the village discharged directly into the burn in which children loved to paddle. No other cases occurred and the exact source of the infection was never discovered.

Disaster

If Morag's case was a diagnostic triumph, the case of young Neil, which occurred a few years later in the same village, illustrates how swiftly disaster can overtaken even the most conscientious diagnostic efforts. In this respect, general practice is a bit like golf; woe to those who, following some isolated triumph, are convinced that they are masters of the game; disaster is for ever round the corner.

Outbreaks of 'summer diarrhoea' are regular visitations in family practice. Several households in the village of Milton had requested visits to their children; symptoms of diarrhoea, tummy pains and occasional vomiting had been relatively mild and recovery swift. I had completed my visits and was preparing to depart for home when I was asked to have a look at Neil in the house up the road.

I prided myself that, by following certain rules, I could gain the confidence of a sick child and carry out an examination in a relaxed atmosphere. (Do anything – chat to Mum, pat the dog, discuss the weather, lift up the doll, rather than directly approach the child, who will thus have time to observe that you don't threaten.) But nothing worked with Neil; he screamed with terror as I entered the kitchen, clung to his mother and tried to hide behind her. His history was similar to that of the other children, most of whom were now recovering from the usual miseries of 'd. and v.' (diarrhoea and vomiting). However gently I tried to approach him, he kicked, struggled and screamed even louder; taking his temperature was almost impossible.

By now I was late, my exasperation was not lessened by Granny, sitting by the fire, who had heralded my arrival with the following announcement to her grandchild, 'Here's the doctor; he'll pit ye in his wee black bag and tak' ye awa,' (no wonder Neil was terrified!), and who, during my vain attempts at examination, kept repeating, 'It's his appendix, doctor; I ken fine it's his appendix.' I longed to reply, 'Oh, please shut up, Granny, I'm the expert here,' but contented myself by reassuring Neil's mother that no treatment apart from saline drinks was called for.

Two days later, being again in the village, I called to see how Neil was getting on; the same screaming resistance again made examination impossible; Granny repeated her pronouncement. One small worry, when we did manage to keep a thermometer in place, was a slight rise in temperature. They called me back two days later; Neil now looked ill, toxic and exhausted. He made no attempt to resist examination; I was appalled to feel a tender swelling over the site of his appendix. They drained the appendix abscess in hospital and to my intense relief he made a complete recovery. I could only apologize to Granny and admit that she had been right and I wrong. There are times when a young GP's lot is not a happy one!

Overconsumption again

In preceding chapters I have tried to explain how, according to

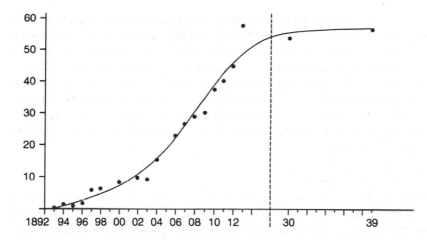

Fig. 10: *Operations for appendicitis at the Edinburgh Royal Infirmary. Appendicectomies are shown per 1000 total admissions between 1892 and 1913. Figures for the years 1899, 1901 and 1905 are not available. (Source: Graph compiled by author from Edinburgh Hospital Reports, Archives Department, Royal Infirmary, Edinburgh.)*

Cleave's theory, overconsumption causes diabetes, obesity and coronary thrombosis. These diseases demonstrate a widespread or generalised effect on the human body of a diet loaded with refined carbohydrates; appendicitis is a localised effect of the same fault. In seeking the cause of acute appendicitis, the history of the appearance of this acute abdominal emergency in the closing decade of the nineteenth century and its dramatic rise in the early decades of the twentieth, is obviously an important clue (see fig. 10).

> When a disease leaps in to extreme prominence within a decade or two, becomes an everyday occurrence in hospitals of certain more civilized countries, and leaves the rest of the world alone, surely the riddle of its causation should not be hard to read.

Thus, in 1920, wrote Rendle Short, a Bristol surgeon, in the opening paragraph of his article, 'The causation of appendicitis'.[1] He concluded that the most likely cause for the appearance of this new disease was 'the relatively less quantity of cellulose eaten on account of the wider use of imported foods'. Short gave impressive evidence from many countries of the two outstanding features of appendicitis; firstly, its

1. A. Rendle Short, 'The causation of appendicitis', *British Journal of Surgery*, vol. 8 (1920), pp. 171–88

extreme rarity or complete absence in 'primitive' societies; secondly, its appearance in Europe in the last decade of the nineteenth century.

We have seen how some doctors tended to confuse the issue by propounding theories about the supposed stressful effects of new inventions (the telephone, the bicycle, etc.) to explain the appearance of appendicitis. But in the last twenty years, the writings of Cleave,[2] Burkitt and others seem to have achieved widespread agreement with Rendle Short that the true explanation for the appearance of appendicitis was dietary.

Conflicting theories

The detailed mechanism explaining why refined carbohydrate should cause the appendix to become acutely inflamed was the subject of disagreement between Cleave and Burkitt. Burkitt stated in 1971[3] that since lack of fibre in modern food was always associated with high sugar consumption, it was difficult to decide which of these faults was the cause; later he appeared to change his mind when he wrote 'lack of dietary fibre is the only adequate explanation of the cause of appendicitis'.[4] He explained the appearance of the disease in the last decade of the nineteenth century by the introduction of steel roller mills for the production of white flour in the 1870s.[5]

Burkitt's change of mind would presumably allow producers of high fibre breakfast cereal to add sugar to their products. But Cleave argued that white flour was being consumed by all classes of people in England by the year 1800 and that most of the fibre contained in wheat bran was by then being removed in sifting in the old stone-grinding mills. Only an additional 6–9 per cent of fibre is removed by steel roller mills. If lack of fibre, arising through the mass consumption of white bread, caused appendicitis, then the disease would have appeared at the beginning, not at the end, of the nineteenth century.

Towards the end of the nineteenth century, sugar consumption had reached unprecedented levels of about 100 lb per caput annually (see fig. 11). Swallowing refined sugar on this scale had, according to Cleave, a profound effect on the bacteria which in their thousands of millions inhabit the human gut. In particular, unabsorbed sugar in the bowel encouraged the growth of Escherichia coli, an organism capable of causing localised inflammation and abscess formation. Other organ-

2. T. L. Cleave, *The Saccharine Disease* (Bristol, John Wright, 1974), p. 120
3. D. P. Burkitt, 'The Aetiology of Appendicitis'. *British Journal of Surgery,* 58, no. 9 (1971), pp. 695–99
4. D. P. Burkitt, *Don't Forget the Fibre in your Diet* (London, Martin Denz, 1979), p. 55
5. Lord Horder, C. Dodds and T. Moran, *Bread* (London, Constable, 1954)

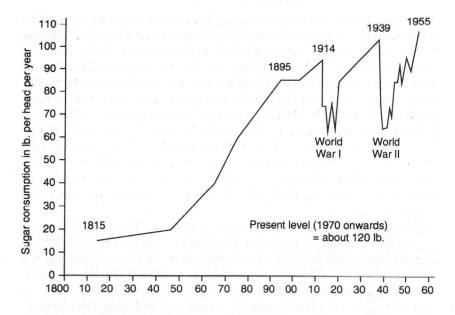

Fig. 11: *The rise in sugar consumption in the UK 1800–1960*
(Source: T. L. Cleave, 'The neglect of natural principles in current medical practice',
Journal of the Royal Naval Medical Service, *vol. XLII no. 2)*

isms allied to E. coli are probably involved; the upshot is abnormal decomposition of food residues in the bowel and an increased tendency to localised bowel infections, including appendicitis. A change from white flour to wholewheat will help to correct constipation, but if Cleave's teaching is correct, unless sugar consumption is at the same time drastically reduced, appendicitis will not be prevented.

In this corner of my dietary wilderness, we need not worry too much whether the cause of appendicitis is lack of fibre in white flour or the disturbing effect on bowel bacteria of excessive sugar. As in the prevention of other manifestations of refined carbohydrate disease, we need only be careful to replace white flour with wholewheat and to try and avoid eating refined sugar altogether.

More confusion

The arrival of a new disease, appendicitis, in the last decade of the nineteenth century, as described by Short and agreed by Cleave, Burkitt and others, did not, however, go undisputed. Some doctors argued then, and still do argue, that the appearance of appendicitis and its rise in the first three decades of the twentieth century reflected nothing but the recognition of a disease which had been there all the time; the operation by Sir Frederick Treves for the removal of the inflamed appendix of King Edward VII just before his coronation, so the theory goes, brought the disease into prominence;[6] only then did doctors begin to recognise it. Well-documented evidence refutes this belief. Short made a detailed study of the records of the Bristol Royal Infirmary and wrote 'Pressure on the Infirmary beds in those days (before 1900) was not so severe; plenty of cases of syphilis, colic, bronchitis, and other mild conditions were admitted. Surely a great number of poorer folk with perforated appendices would have sought admission if they had existed'.[7]

Hospital records in Edinburgh tell the same story. Joseph Bell, a distinguished surgeon on the staff of Edinburgh Royal Infirmary in the late nineteenth century, was famed as a clinical teacher and for his unique skill in deducing important facts about his patients' background and habits by noting seemingly trivial details of dress or appearance; one of his students, the young Conan Doyle, later immortalised Bell's method in the fictitious Baker Street rooms of Sherlock Holmes and Doctor Watson.

Bell was the first surgeon to be appointed to the staff of the Royal Edinburgh Hospital for Sick Children. In 1893, he issued a report on the previous five years' work in the hospital's surgical wards. Detailed accounts are given of cases of severe burns, of 'most marvellous recoveries' of children who had fallen from buildings onto the spiked tops of iron railings; large numbers of cases of glandular and joint tuberculosis are dealt with, as are cases of hernia and congenital abnormalities. Not one single case of appendicitis is included.[8]

In a companion article to the 1893 report, another surgeon, Alexis Thomson, also working in the Children's Hospital, gives a more detailed account of surgical cases: 'In 90 per cent of cases the child was found to be suffering from one or other of four causes of disease, in the following order of frequency, viz. tuberculosis, sepsis, malformation, rickets. The small minority of 10 per cent were attributable all the other etiological factors combined, e.g. traumatism, syphilis, nerve growths, nerve lesions'. Thomson classified diseases caused by suppuration or sepsis as follows:

6. A. Rendle Short, 'The causation of appendicitis'
7. Ibid
8. Edinburgh Hospital Reports 1893 (Edinburgh, The Royal Infirmary, Archives Department)

a) Local surface infections of skin and mucous membranes
b) Lymphatic glandular infections
c) Middle ear suppuration
d) Suppuration in connection with the skeleton.

Again, appendicitis is not once mentioned.

The case of Neil of Milton village is highly significant in the light of these hospital reports from last century; his case illustrates one outcome of unoperated appendicitis – fever, lassitude, toxaemia and the formation of an abscess. The other outcome is rupture of the inflamed and perhaps gangrenous appendix followed by generalised peritonitis from which the patient rarely survives. Both outcomes, abscess or peritonitis, are marked by prolonged, debilitating illness with fever, pain, vomiting and wasting. It is inconceivable that parents who would readily bring to the hospital children suffering from swollen glands, injuries and so forth, would leave at home their brothers or sisters with suppurating appendices. If the disease occurred in the 1890s on anything like the scale today, it would have appeared in hospital reports.

The absence of a single case of appendicitis (or perityphlitis as it was first known) in the Edinburgh Children's Hospital Reports of 1893 is matched by the absence of a single instance of acute coronary thrombosis in the cases of 'angina pectoris' collected by the late Sir James McKenzie.[9] It is also matched by the well-authenticated statement that duodenal ulcer is a new disease of the twentieth century.[10] I have dwelt at some length on the history of the appearance of these diseases of civilization because, as Rendle Short suggested, the sudden appearance of a new disease in certain populations and its absence in others, surely give a strong clue as to cause.

Confusion again

Unfortunately a multitude of changes occur in the food, habits and environment of primitive rural populations when they migrate to modern cities. McCarrison repeatedly emphasised that in determining patterns of health and disease, the most important of these changes was dietary; he demonstrated how the bowels of laboratory rats became subject to inflammation and degeneration when a diet of whole, fresh, varied food was changed to one of refined flour, processed proteins and fats and much refined sugar. There was strong evidence, he argued, for believing that the same process was at work

9. James MacKenzie, *Angina Pectoris* (London, Henry Frowde and Hodder and Stoughton, 1923)
10. C. W. F. Illingworth, *Peptic Ulcer* (Edinburgh and London, E. & S. Livingstone, 1953) p. 71

in free, living human beings. No case of appendicitis in the Hunza tribe was seen by McCarrison during the nine years he worked as their medical officer.[11]

However compelling the evidence based on relatively simple observations, medical scientists, alas, appear to have a strong urge to spurn the simple outlines and to seek complexity. In the last two years papers have been published whose authors argue that the appearance of appendicitis was due to developments in plumbing technology.[12] According to the new theory, food and water supplies in our nineteenth century cities were so heavily contaminated that citizens were for ever swallowing harmful bacteria and viruses. By constant exposure to infection children built up immunity to attack by certain organisms; this immunity disappeared when modern bathrooms heralded a new era of environmental cleanliness. This theory seems to me to be extremely implausible. The numbers of cases of appendicitis in Edinburgh illustrated in fig. 10 were exactly the same in scale and timing as those from hospitals in Bristol[13] and Oxford.[14] According to the hygiene theory, the scale and timing of plumbing improvements would have to have been the same in the three cities; such uniformity is highly unlikely. Mass production of processed foods and the railway system in operation by the turn of the century ensured that the rising tonnage of sugar and sugar-containing foods were widely and uniformly distributed.

Disease clustering

In seeking the cause of diseases of our time we should not look at any one disease in isolation; if diseases of different bodily systems begin to appear at the same time, often in the same patient, and if evidence points to a profound change in dietary habits, it is reasonable to suppose that all the diseases may have a common dietary cause.

My diagram (Fig 12) attempts to illustrate Cleave's explanation of the appearance of the four manifestations of what he called the 'Saccharine disease' during this century. The existence of an 'incubation period' is crucial to our understanding of the timing of the appearance of the various diseases. Cleave suggested that as soon as the consumption of refined sugar approached 100 lb per head of population a 'fuse' was lighted; the 'explosion' of appendicitis occurred immediately, of

11. R. McCarrison, 'Faulty Food in relation to Gastro-Intestinal Disease', *Journal of the American Medical Association*, 78, no. 1 (1922), p. 2
12. K. W. Heaton 'Aetiology of acute appendicitis', *BMJ*, 294 (1987) pp. 1632–3
13. A. Rendle Short, 'The causation of appendicitis'
14. T. L. Cleave, *The Saccharine Disease*, p. 126

A ken fine it's his appendix

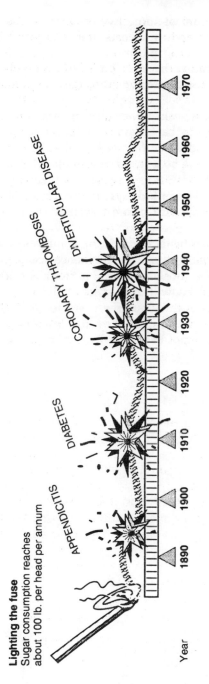

Fig. 12: *T. L. Cleave's incubation period fuse*
(Source: author, based on Cleave's concept)

137

diabetes after a minimum of some twenty years, of coronary thrombosis after thirty years and of diverticular disease after forty years. These figures are averages; enormous variations exist both in the amount of sugar consumed by individuals and in their susceptibility to disease, but where records are available, they confirm the incubation period.

One last thing must be said about any disease caused by invasion of any part of the body by bacteria; the virulence of, as far as I know, all bacteria can wax and wane for reasons that are not clear. Scarlet fever, which follows attack by a strain of bacteria called a streptococcus was still regarded in the 1930s as a serious notifiable disease because of its complications in heart or kidneys. Today scarlet fever has become a trivial affair, a mild transient throat infection; often the scarlet rash is hardly detectable.

Although acute appendicitis remains the commonest surgical emergency in British hospitals today, the incidence has steadily declined since the 1930s. Maybe those invading bacteria are losing some of their vigour; we do not know; but in spite of all the arguments about hygiene, I remain convinced that if we are to prevent this serious abdominal emergency we should obey the teaching of Cleave and McCarrison. The fault is not in our baths, but in our food.

19 The Scourge of Coronary Thrombosis

A GP living 'over the shop' enjoys the convenience of being able to slip through to his desk in the evening and to tie up the loose ends of the day that has passed or to prepare for the day ahead. But this convenience carries the seed of trouble; the workaholic tends never to leave his work and to isolate himself from his family; his profession takes over so much of his life that he tends to lose his sense of balance and so becomes a less competent doctor. During the first fifteen years of our life in Aberfeldy, when my wife and I occupied the cornershop which is now the central practice premises, we became increasingly aware of this conflict between the demands of work and of family. Another disadvantage, from the doctor's point of view, lay in the opportunity seized by patients who, on seeing the surgery light on, would blithely ring the night bell and say: 'I saw you were in, doctor, and wondered if you could renew my prescription'. This carefree attitude to a doctor's time is one unfortunate consequence of a 'free' health service.

But as I sat writing on this quiet autumn evening in the corner consulting room, there was no doubt about the urgency in the running footsteps thumping on the pavement, and in the hectic ringing of the night bell. 'Come quickly to the Town Hall, doctor, Alec's collapsed; he's terribly ill.' The badminton club players, scared and hushed, stood in small groups around the court where Alec lay, dead; he could not be resuscitated. He had just finished a game and collapsed while talking to his companions.

Alec, in his forties, played championship tennis in the summer; in winter he kept fit by playing energetic badminton. He was one of a long list of athletes whose pursuit of physical fitness did not protect them from coronary disease of the heart (CDH). These sad cases contradict studies, published from time to time in the medical press, which seem to demonstrate that those whose work involves hard physical toil suffer less from CDH than do men in sedentary occupations.

If hard exercise gives any protection from this modern heart disease, gamekeepers, farmers and shepherds would suffer very little; Highland practices such as ours would see few cases. But CDH seems to be no less common among rural workers living in this peaceful Highland glen than among those who toil in the rush and din of the city. In 1971 I made a few informal inquiries on the frequency of coronary thrombosis in other practices in the Highlands; all the doctors whom I questioned confirmed regular encounters with this disease. Dr Fergusson of Beauly, in Inverness-shire, with a practice list of 1,500, told me that in the month of August 1971 he had seen nine new cases, all of whom resided in his practice area. If physical exercise plays any role in preventing CDH, it must be very small. Does the craze for jogging do more harm than good? Do the strained muscles, tendons, joints and even broken bones which appear to afflict the jogger, as he or she pounds along hard pavements, cancel any benefit? The agonised expressions during the jogging ritual do not speak of relaxation or of pleasure!

What a heavy load of sorrow, hardship and anguish falls on the widows of men struck down by CDH before their time; the terrible task of going to Alec's wife as she sat by her fire, to tell her that her husband was dead, had to be faced; how can words be found? Can there be any more stressful thing to do in all general practice than this?

Vivid memories of tragic coronary incidents underline the urgency of knowing the cause and seeking prevention. I tried to put myself in Mrs McKenzie's shoes as I left her house and stood wearily for a moment on the doorstep and listened to the waves of the loch breaking on the stony shore. A strong west wind sent moonlit clouds racing above the hills on the other side of the loch. 'He woke up about four o'clock with this terrible pain in his chest. I went through to the kitchen to make him a cup of tea and when I came back with the cup, he was silent and I saw he was dead.' He had been out at his work as a gamekeeper on the previous day, with no hint of trouble – out as usual on long patrols of hill and forest.

In January 1968 one of the worst gales of the century swept across central Scotland. It was probably not quite as severe as the gale of October 1987 in southern England, but the damage was extensive and. severe. In Glasgow, roofs, slates and chimneys went flying and, as if by some giant's scythe, wide stretches of forest were laid flat in the path of the storm. By now, with our family of two boys and one girl, we had moved from the crossroads to the Dorran bungalow we had been able to build by the Urlar road. The house, which stands exposed to the full force of a south-westerly gale on a small wooded hill, shook and rattled during the night and felt as if at any moment it might take off. Awful destruction was seen in the morning. All that remained of a little summerhouse was splintered glass and wood, strewn among the oak trees, and the trees themselves had suffered; some were toppled and others leaning, partly uprooted.

In the months that followed, contractors had to be brought in to clear up the mess and to fell trees thought to be unsafe. By December, the place was beginning to look less like a battlefield; the final felling of three trees by the gate had been entrusted to Duncan. Duncan, aged forty-eight, worked a small hill farm and like so many in his shoes had to augment his income outside farming. He had started contracting for timber felling; often, his wife helped him in this work.

Having attended her at the births of their three children I knew the family well. Duncan was a cheerful, enterprising man with an inventive turn of mind; gifted with considerable engineering skill, he had improved on several types of farm machinery; he was also an artist whose paintings showed no mean talent. Some months previously, when he consulted me because of transient backache, I had been struck by his superb physical fitness. He appeared to enjoy the hard challenge of his work, and with his hobbies and stable family seemed to be one of those people perfectly suited to the life and work they have chosen.

So it was with some surprise that, while doing visits in the town before lunch on a December morning, I received an urgent message to go at once to my house where Duncan had collapsed. I found him crouched in his Land-Rover, his wife doing her best to comfort him. Ashen pale to the lips, he told of crippling pain across his chest radiating down both his arms.

The classic symptoms and signs of coronary thrombosis make this disease, with few exceptions, one of the easiest to diagnose in general practice. In a case such as this, confirmation by electrocardiograph or blood enzyme estimation seemed hardly necessary; they were, of course, done and confirmed the diagnosis when he was admitted to the cottage hospital.

Tragic procession.
Duncan is another example of the tragic multitude of Scotland's CDH victims – our country has the distinction of being near the top of the world league of coronary deaths. Some sufferers make good recoveries and return to full activity; others are not so fortunate. Duncan did recover and was able to go back to work; but, sad to relate, he suffered another attack some eighteen months later from which he did not recover. One estimate of the frequency of coronary thrombosis states:

> In an average general practice there are 500 male patients between 34 and 64, about 100 of which are likely to have coronary attacks before retiring age. Of these, 25 will die suddenly before medical aid can be called, a further 15 will not survive the initial episode.[1]

As well as the anguish of bereavement in family life, this toll of disability and death brings a serious drain on the reservoirs of male skill and experience (coronary heart disease is far less common in premenopausal women than in men). The victims of coronary thrombosis are often at an age of maximum usefulness to their families and nation.

What is the cause?
As more and more deaths from coronary disease of the heart began to be recorded in western nations in the 1950s, the need to find the cause and the means of prevention became urgent. The mountain of scientific papers on this subject is now too vast for any one explorer to climb. Here is the wilderness of claim and counter-claim, mentioned in my introduction.

Our path through the wilderness will be clarified if we remember the following three features of CDH which must be in accord with any theory of causation.

1 History. Like duodenal ulcer, coronary thrombosis – the sudden heart attack coming out of the blue, in men in their forties, fifties and sixties – is a new disease of the twentieth century. On this there is wide agreement. Dr Rae Gilchrist, a former Honorary consulting physician

1. K. P. Ball, 'The aetiology of coronary artery disease', *Update*, 16, vol. 5 (1978), pp. 521–9

at the Royal Infirmary in Edinburgh, recorded the first case in Scotland in 1928. He had read reports in American literature of a new phenomenon, sudden blockage of the coronary arteries, and wrote: 'I had never previously heard of coronary thrombosis even though I had four years post-graduate experience and my Membership examination behind me.'[2]

Dr Gilchrist gives the account of cases in his wards as follows:

Years	No. of cases	Period
1924–26	0	2 years
1928–30	12	2 years
1939–46	100	7 years
1947–54	321	7 years[3]

By the 1970s over 500 cases annually were being admitted to the coronary care unit of the Edinburgh Royal Infirmary.[4]

My former neighbour, the late Dr Jack Henderson (1900–79) of Pitlochry, whose special interest was heart disease, stated in a lecture delivered in 1964: 'In 1925 coronary thrombosis was a rare disease and I do not recall seeing *even one example* of it when I was a student'[5] (author's italics). Dr Henderson's student days were spent in Glasgow, now regarded as one of the world's coronary headquarters. I have elsewhere tried to show why these findings cannot possibly be explained by supposing that the physicians of those days, even without the diagnostic methods of modern medicine, were unable to recognise coronary thrombosis.[6]

The appearance of coronary thrombosis in the 1920s rules out genetic factors as of any importance. Human genetic make-up cannot alter in the course of a few decades; the causes therefore must be environmental, a fact which does not conflict with the tendency of CDH to run in families. Familial clustering of this degenerative disease simply means that owing to their individual make-up, some people are more prone than others to succumb to a harmful environment; but it is the harmful environment (in this case, dietary), not genetic weakness, that makes them ill. It follows that something profoundly

2 Rae Gilchrist, 'Edinburgh tradition in clinical cardiology', *Scottish Medical Journal*, vol. 17, no. 248 (1972)

3. Rae Gilchrist, personal communication to author, 1971

4. R. M. Marquis, Smith, Kline and French Cardiovascular Forum (Swan Press, 1979)

5. J. Henderson, 'Looking back to McKenzie', *Journal of the Royal College of General Practitioners*, 7 (1964), pp. 9–23

6. W. W. Yellowlees, 'Sir James McKenzie and the history of myocardial infarction', *Journal of Royal College of General Practitioners*, 32 (1982) pp. 109–12

harmful in our dietary environment must have happened towards the end of the nineteenth century.

2. *Dangerous trade routes.* Isolated peoples still living outside the trade routes of what we call civilization do not suffer from CDH, but when they emigrate to or are engulfed by 'civilization' their coronary arteries become diseased.[7]

3. *Disease clustering.* Where coronary thrombosis is common, so is obesity and diabetes;[8] often these three conditions occur in the same individual, a phenomenon which follows the mechanism of overconsumption.

To sum up: I have argued that neither a lack of physical exercise nor the presence of urban-type stress can be important causes of CDH; in the following two chapters I shall point a finger at the aspect of civilization which I believe is the basic dietary cause of this twentieth-century scourge – the unprecedented rise, in the second half of the nineteenth century, in the consumption of sugar.

7. A. M. Cohen, S. Bavly and R. Poznanksi, 'Changes in Diet in Yemeni Jews in relation to Diabetes and Ischaemic Heart Disease', *The Lancet*, 7217, vol. 2 (1961), pp. 1399–1401
8. T. L. Cleave, *The Saccharine Disease* (Bristol, John Wright, 1974), p. 107

20 Coronary Thrombosis: Fats Ancient and Modern

Tobacco, especially cigarette smoking, is given a prominent place as one of the risk factors of coronary disease of the heart (CDH). Studies in this country have repeatedly shown higher incidence and death rates among heavy smokers. But national comparisons do not confirm tobacco as a basic cause. The citizens of Japan, Switzerland, the Netherlands and Sweden all smoke more heavily than do the British, yet they have lower (and in Japan, far lower) death rates from heart disease.[1] As in our experience of lung cancer, the very high numbers of deaths in Scotland cannot be explained only by cigarette smoking; there must be some other factor which makes our Scottish population more prone than other nations to CDH and to cancer.

If lack of exercise, cigarette-smoking or stress are merely secondary, and not basic causes of CDH, what then is the basic cause? What has happened to what we call the 'advanced' nations of the human race to cause this twentieth-century epidemic of heart disease; what aspect of civilisation brings disease to the hitherto healthy coronary arteries of 'primitive' peoples who live outside the trade routes of the West?

Fashionable fats

The fashionable answer to this question is that our cardiac downfall is caused by our liking for dietary fats, especially saturated fats, which are found in dairy produce and in the butcher's shop. In the UK, we are said on average to get 40 per cent or more of our energy from dietary fat; a spate of official reports tell us that this figure is too high and that it should be reduced to 35 per cent or less.[2]

---

1. M. Wynn and A. Wynn, *Prevention of Handicap and Health of Women* (London, Routledge and Kegan Paul, 1979), p 87
2. *The Health of the Nation* (London, HMSO, 1991)

The coronary arteries of victims of CDH are studded with fatty deposits; these deposits which usually include a fat called cholesterol, when covered by a thrombus, or clot, may ultimately block the artery and so induce a heart attack; the whole process, in medical terminology, is called 'arteriosclerosis'. In the 1950s, extension of laboratory facilities made possible more frequent blood cholesterol estimations and it seemed that people with raised blood cholesterol levels were more prone to coronary attacks. Soon the following sequence was accepted far and wide as the explanation for the coronary scourge:

Saturated fats → high blood cholesterol → arteriosclerosis → coronary thrombosis.

Fats, found in animal or vegetable tissues, are made up of collections of fatty acids which, according to their molecular make-up, are termed saturated or unsaturated; saturated fatty acids, got mostly from animal products, are solid at room temperature, while unsaturated oils from vegetables or fish remain liquid. This is no place for biochemical detail; suffice it to say that when fatty acids have an enhanced quality of unsaturation they are known as polyunsaturated fats; when the latter are substituted for saturated fats they (polyunsaturates) can often lower the level of blood cholesterol.

By the 1960s, on both sides of the Atlantic physicians had become so enthusiastic about the fat theory of the cause of CDH that dietary regimes in which polyunsaturated fats were substituted for traditional animal fats became the order of the day. Committees were formed; campaigns with government backing were launched. Butter, beef, whole milk and eggs became the villains of modern nutrition. The margarine industry quickly seized the chance of undreamed-of expansion if housewives, obsessed with blood cholesterol levels, could be persuaded to replace butter by polyunsaturated margarine and lard by vegetable cooking oils. By 1980 the commercial success of this policy was seen in a review in Aberdeen which found on supermarket shelves reserved for fats only some 20 per cent of space left for butter; margarines or shortening made from 'pure vegetable oils' occupied the rest.[3] The following figures give some idea of the costs of advertising processed oils and margarines compared with what is spent on promoting natural butter.

---

3. E. Smith, 'Atherogenicity and the Supermarket Shelf', *The Lancet*, 8167, vol. 1 (1980), p534

Table 2: *Purchase of butter, margarine and spreads*

	1975	1987
Butter	£1.6 million	£ 8.3 million
Margarine	£2.6 million	£11.5 milion
Spreads (low/mixed)		£20.1 million

(Source: Media Expenditure Analysis Ltd)

(In passing, please note that the above figures pale into insignificance when compared with the £100 million lavished on advertising by the sugar industry.[4])

The scare of animal fats, based entirely on biochemical theory, is unimpressive to those guided by commonsense and by a knowledge of dietary history. Nor would it impress followers of Cleave or McCarrison who believe that human beings are adapted to foods as they occur in nature.

Ancestral diets

Since the very dawn of human evolution our prehistoric ancestors have lived off the flesh and fat of animals. The dramatic paintings by Palaeolithic hunters seen in the caves of southern France give us a glimpse of the dependence of these people on animal foods.

> In view of the climatic conditions prevailing in the Ice Age when the pictures (on the cave walls) were made it is clear that our ancestors of this epoch must have relied solely upon game as their food . . . each Ice Age lasted between 50,000 and 100,000 years.[5]

Thus wrote Dr Wolfgang Lutz of Salzburg who suffered from chronic dyspepsia, dental decay and crippling pain in his hip joints and who, as he admired the cave paintings, wondered if we were not primarily adapted to an ancestral diet of animal flesh and fat; within a very short time of starting a four-year trial of eating only animal proteins and fats – no carbohydrate at all – the good doctor noted a remarkable improvement in wellbeing and complete resolution of his dental, digestive and joint troubles. During the last thirty years, he reckons that he has successfully treated more than ten thousand patients by advising a protein-fat diet, modified by experience to include 70 grams (about 2 ounces) of carbohydrate daily. The regime, claims Dr Lutz,

4. J. Yudkin, *Pure White and Deadly* (London, Penguin Books, 1986), p162
5. Wolfgang Lutz, *Dismantling a Myth: The Role of Fat and Carbohydrate in our Diet* (Springfield, Chas. Thomas, 1986)

is particularly effective for patients suffering from digestive ailments including Crohn's Disease.

Abundant evidence exists in ancient writings, including the Old Testament, of the widespread use of dairy produce; Neolithic ceramic cheese-strainers found in Mesopotamia, Greece and Crete confirm the antiquity of milk and its products as much-desired foods of mankind.[6]

Are we really to believe that these traditional fats, prized for their taste and health-giving qualities, could at the beginning of the twentieth century suddenly become the cause of catastrophic death and disability? And are we to agree that the integrity of our hearts depends on our buying and consuming a fancy brand of margarine? The following observations among diverse races suggests that the answer is emphatically 'NO'.

1. Studies among East African Masai and Samburu tribes, who get about 60 per cent of their calories from meat, blood or milk, revealed remarkable freedom from coronary disease.[7]

2. In Israel, immigrants arriving from the Yemen, whose dietary fat in their native habitat had come from beef, mutton and butter were found to be free from CDH and diabetes.[8]

3. Icelanders, who in the nineteenth century got about 80–85 per cent of their calories from proteins and fats, did not suffer at all from diabetes; the same freedom from this disease had been recorded among the Eskimos.[9]

4. From the novels of Dickens, and from studies by Rowntree,[10] we can be sure that in Britain during the nineteenth century the wealthy, servant-keeping classes ate enormously of animal fats, but they did not suffer from coronary thrombosis.

5. The commonest source of dietary cholesterol is egg yolk; but the level of cholesterol in our blood is determined, not by the number of eggs which we eat, but by the body's own internal mechanism centered in the liver; surely we must assume that cholesterol plays a vital protective role in bodily transactions.

6. D. and P. Brothwell, *Food in Antiquity* (London, Thames and Hudson, 1969), p59
7. 'The Masai's Cholesterol', *BMJ* Leading Article, 5769 (1971), pp 262–3
8. A. M. Cohen and others, 'Changes in the Diet of Yemeni Jews in Relation to Diabetes and Heart Disease', *The Lancet*, 7217, vol. 2 (1961), pp. 1399–1401
9. T. L. Cleave, *The Saccharine Disease* (Bristol, John Wright, 1974), p90
10. L. Michaels, 'The Aetiology of Coronary Heart Disease', *British Heart Journal*, vol. 28 (1966), p261

The Industrial Revolution

The late Lord Boyd-Orr, in his book *Food and the People*,[11] outlined the change in the British diet which came with the industrial revolution:

> The diet of the (working class) people consisted mainly of wheaten bread, oatmeal, potatoes, milk, butter, cheese and vegetables. These are all protective foods, rich in essential minerals and vitamins ... As the industrial towns grew in size, the quality of the diet deteriorated. Milk, dairy products and vegetables, which were cheap in the country, were expensive in the towns. There was a change-over from wholemeal bread, rich in vitamins, to white flour which is poor in vitamins. The consumption of oatmeal fell. The consumption of refined sugar, which has neither vitamins nor minerals, rose from a few pounds per head per annum in the beginning of the nineteenth century to nearly a hundredweight per head by the end of the century. Hence the diet of the working class came to consist mainly of cheap energy yielding foods, poor in both vitamins and minerals.

The change from natural fresh food to processed foods including white flour, margarine and sugar resulted in widespread nutritional deficiency, in stunted stature and disease in the poorer classes of our industrial cities; and the huge increase in sugar consumption by the end of the century, as Cleave has demonstrated, lit the fuse which in the 1920s and 1930s was to activate the coronary explosion.

Incoming Sugar Tide

By the 1960s, observations throughout the world had shown a similar pattern of events wherever rising sugar consumption approached 100 lb. per head per annum; the Yemeni immigrants in Israel, the Icelanders and Eskimos mentioned above, and other races detailed by Cleave, all developed diabetes and coronary thrombosis as they changed from animal foods to refined flour and sugar.

In Natal, South Africa, settlers from India who arrived during the last century to work in sugar plantations now suffer far higher rates of diabetes and coronary thrombosis than Indians dwelling in the regions of India whence the settlers came. Again the change in their diet features a ninefold increase in sugar intake and an increase in the use of unsaturated vegetable oils. In his studies of the high incidence of diabetes among the Natal Indians, Dr G. D. Campbell has found

---

11. J. Boyd Orr, *Food and the People* (London, Pilot Press, 1943), p15

that, compared with other races, Indians seem to be more susceptible to arterial disease associated with diabetes.[12]

Their higher susceptibility would explain why a review of death rates from coronary thrombosis in the London districts of Harrow and Brent found that Asians (mostly from the Indian subcontinent) suffered higher rates of coronary disease than Europeans living in those same London districts; yet those Asians smoked less than Europeans, consumed less cholesterol and less saturated fat and ate far more unsaturated vegetable oil (mostly corn oil) and more fibre.[13]

Fats in Europe

In Europe, no constant relationship can be found between animal fat consumption and heart disease. Countries like France or Switzerland, where the per caput intake of animal fats is higher than or similar to the UK, have lower death rates from CDH. An average Frenchman or Frenchwoman consumes 42 grammes of dairy fat per day, compared with 28.8 grammes in Britain, yet the coronary death rate in France is almost one quarter that of the rate in England and Wales.[14] The following table constructed by A. Barfield, an agricultural scientist, shows how 'all countries (except Finland) which eat more fat, or a higher proportion of animal fat, have lower levels of coronary heart disease than does Britain'.[15]

The failure to find any relationship between saturated fat consumption and mortality from CDH in European countries was confirmed in a 1988 WHO Regional Publication (European series No. 24, Copenhagen). The authors of this study, however, give the incomprehensible advice that their failure to find such a relationship should not refute their belief that the relationship does exist![16] Does this example of biased reporting remove all hope of finding objective statements even in WHO publications? Does it confirm a depressing conversation I was recently privileged to have with a very distinguished nutritionist who told me of his fear that WHO was sometimes being used as a front for commercial interests?

---

12 T. L. Cleave and G. D. Campbell, *Diabetes, Coronary Thrombosis and the Saccharine Disease* (Bristol, John Wright & Sons, 1969)

13. McKeigue and others, 'Diet and Risk Factors in Asians in North West London', *The Lancet*, 8464, vol. 2 (1985), pp 1086–90

14. G. Segel, 'Autres Pays, Autres Moeurs', *BMJ*, vol. 29 (1989), pp 83–85

15. A. Barfield, 'Food and Health Policy', *The Lancet*, 8511, vol. 1 (1980), p 534

16. W. P. T. James and others, *Healthy Nutrition: preventing nutrition related diseases in Europe* (Copenhagen, WHO Regional Office for Europe, 1988)

Table 3:   *Fat supplies and death rates in certain European countries and USA*

Country	Total fat*	Energy from animal fat‡	CDH death rate+
Netherlands	183	31.8	165.4
Belgium	179	30.3	155.1
Denmark	172	34.5	181.7
USA	168	25.2	217.8
Switzerland	168	29.4	96.1
France	157	28.0	73.0
Austria	156	26.8	160.5
Sweden	149	30.9	159.1
West Germany	143	26.3	150.4
United Kingdom**	142	27.4	262.6
Eire	141	25.8	258.0
Finland	131	31.0	314.2
Spain	128	17.2	82.5

(Source: *The Lancet*, 8511, Vol. 2 (1986), Letters, p. 868)
*Total fat grammes per head per day 1978–81 (source FAO)
‡Energy from animal fat as percentage of total calories 1978–9 (source FAO)
+Deaths from ischaemic heart disease in men aged 45–54 per 100,000 (source WHO 1980)
**England and Wales

Milk cows in the Highlands

Until the 1920s, before coronary thrombosis had been heard of, and within the memory of many of my former elderly patients, morning and evening milking were part of the rhythm of life in the Highlands of Scotland. Many of the main street houses in Aberfeldy had cow byres and a laddie was employed to take the cows daily to their common grazing ground. Butter and cheese were produced locally in abundance. The dependence of the Highlander on his cows followed a long tradition:

> 'It was said in the early 1600s that the Highlanders, who lived solely on milk, cheese and flesh, were able to supply cheese to the Lowlands at times when cereals were scarce there'.[17]

Mass produced margarine began to appear in our shops at the end of the nineteenth century; if dietary fats are to be blamed as the cause of coronary thrombosis margarine is a far more likely culprit than butter.[18]

Stall-feeding

Enthusiasts for polyunsaturated margarine respond to this defence of

---

17. A. Fenton, *Country Life in Scotland: Our Rural Past* (Edinburgh, J. Donald, 1987), p154
18. W. Martin, 'Margarine, not Butter the Culprit', *The Lancet*, vol. 2 (1983), p407

traditional fats by blaming modern agricultural practices for altering the quality and quantity of animal fats in domestic animals. In particular they attack the fattening of cattle by stall feeding.[19] This argument has been completely demolished by Cleave (*The Saccharine Disease* pp. 102–3), who reminds us of the value of animal fats in giving flavour to meat and of the selective breeding which traditionally was geared to evolving fat animals.

For centuries the Swiss, with their relatively low rate of CDH mortality, have stall-fed their animals during snow-bound Alpine winters. Moreover, Cleave points out that without the use of modern machinery and modern chemical solvents, the vegetable oils, derived from cotton seed, maize, soya bean and rapeseed, would be unavailable for human food. These unnatural fats are extracted from the crushed seeds by the use of powered presses or toxic solvents, traces of which remain in the finished product. Repeated heating to very high temperatures ensures a stable odourless product, and finally butylated hydroxyanisole is added as an antioxidant.[20] Such processing alters the molecular structure of the supposedly beneficial polyunsaturated vegetable oils; the long-term effect on human beings who consume this alien, unnatural food is unknown; cholesterol blood levels may be reduced, but the change from butter and animal fat to new processed vegetable oils has failed completely to demonstrate any improvement in death rates.

Olive and palm

The charge of 'unnatural food' cannot be made against the oil extracted widely in Mediterranean countries from the flesh of the olive or against the palm oil, beloved by Pacific islanders and by peoples in many parts of Africa. Both these vegetable oils can be extracted from the parent plant by simple technologies dependent on human or animal muscle power; their use as human food does not require sophisticated machinery nor complex processing; like dairy produce, they have been the food of mankind since the dawn of history.

Official spokesmen and media pundits often advise us that we should adopt a Mediterranean diet so that our CDH death rates will approach the relatively low levels of southern European countries, Greece, Portugal, Italy and Spain. They do so because of the belief that the cardiac health of the peoples of these countries is due to their dependence on vegetable oil and their liking for fresh fruits and vegetables. Why do these advisers never remind us that populations

19. M. Crawford, 'Prevention of Coronary Disease', *BMJ*, 6024, vol. 1 (1976), p1532
20. R. H. Hall *Food for Naught* (New York and London, Harper Row, 1974), p235

who have access to an abundance of their own fresh fruits and vegetables usually eat less sugar (see the table below); thus the relative freedom of these southern Europeans from CDH confirms excessive sugar consumption as the most likely cause of the disease.

Table 4: *Consumption of centrifugal sugar by countries, pre-war average and 1958*

Country	Pre-war	Kilograms per caput	1958
UK	49.0		52.8
Greece	11.1		12.6
Portugal	10.0		16.4
Italy	7.9		19.4
Spain	12.4		16.5

(Source: FAO Publications, Rome 1961)

The pre-war and 1958 figures for sugar consumption are important because of the thirty-year incubation period which elapses between the time when the annual per caput intake reaches 40 kilograms (90–100lb) and the explosion of CDH.

Since 1958 Portugal's intake has risen to 32 kilograms, Spain's to 24 (1987 figures); unfortunately, the Sugar Year Book no longer publishes per caput sugar consumption for individual European countries; only EEC averages are given. It remains to be seen whether trends in tourism, trade and agriculture in southern Europe will bring a level of sugar consumption to match that of Britain. If that day comes and if, as I believe, Cleave's thesis is true, then the men of Greece, Portugal, Italy and Spain will lose their relative freedom from the scourge of coronary deaths.

Japan often shares the role of southern European countries as a shining example of very low death rates from CDH. Again I must ask, why do the evangelists for prevention of coronary disease never mention Japan's apparently very low per caput sugar consumption?

Table 5: *Sugar consumption by UK and Japan*

	Kilograms per caput per annum		
	Pre-war average	1958	1987
UK	49 kg	52 kg	37.8 kg*
Japan	12.3 kg	13.7 kg	22.1 kg

(Source: FAO Publications, Rome, 1961: Sugar Year Book, London, 1987)
*The true UK consumption is probably over 40 kg; only EEC averages seem to be available

In this chapter, I have tried to argue firstly that on grounds of history, epidemiology and commonsense, the dietary fat theory of the cause of CDH cannot be sustained; and secondly that the evidence incriminating refined carbohydrate, especially sugar, although far more convincing, has been neglected and forgotten. My views on dietary fats are not the ravings of a lone rural GP; distinguished medical scientists – Ahrens, Harper, Mann, Olson, Brisson in North America, and in Europe McMichael, Oliver, Mitchell, McCormick, Skrabanaek and Dedichen, have argued forcibly against the theory that CDH can be prevented by changes in fat consumption. The role of refined sugar has been elaborated by Cleave, Yudkin, Frohnm, Vickery and Aykroyd; but neither in Europe nor in America have these men evidently found favour in the corridors of power, a fact which is all the more remarkable in view of the total failure which I shall attempt to outline in the next chapter, to detect any improvement in death rates when the fat theory is put into practice. As we shall see, in some trials, substituting vegetable oils for animal fats appears to have increased rather than improved death rates.

21 Cholesterol and The Censorship of Fashion

In 1956 Norway launched one of the earliest attempts on a national scale to prevent CDII by reducing dietary fat consumption and by substituting soya oil and margarine for butter. In reviewing the programme some twenty years later Dr Jens Dedichen deplored the fact that many Norwegians had become so obsessed with blood cholesterol levels that they had been turned into nervous wrecks;[1] he pointed out that the campaign, far from preventing CDH, had been followed by a steep and continuing rise in death rates from heart attacks; the rising curve of coronary deaths bore a remarkable resemblance to that of increasing consumption of soya oil! Did this vegetable oil have a toxic effect on the coronary arteries? When Dr Dedichen voiced his concern at this failure of a dietary prevention programme, he was surprised at the hostile reaction of his colleagues: 'I was quite simply accused of being ignorant. Worse, I was censored'.

A trial, similar in outline to Norway's, carried out from St Mary's Hospital, London,[2] also ended in failure. Patients attending with signs of coronary disease were divided into three groups, two of which were treated by a cut in their consumption of milk, butter and eggs and a switch to olive oil for one group and corn oil for the other. The third group, untreated as a control, continued their usual diet. At the end of two years, when results were assessed, the lowest mortality was recorded in the third untreated group; the *highest* mortality occurred in the corn oil group, that is the only group in the trial whose blood cholesterol levels had been significantly lowered. The exercise, there-

1. J. Dedichen, 'Cholesterol and Atherosclerosis Once More', *Journal of the Norwegian Medical Association*, no. 16 (1976), pp. 915–19
2. G. A. Rose, and others, 'Corn Oil in Treatment of Ischaemic Heart Disease', *BMJ*, 5449, vol. 1 (1965), pp. 1531–33

fore, could hardly be described as a triumph for a cholesterol-lowering regime; but enthusiasts for polyunsaturated fats, undeterred, suggested that if cholesterol-lowering was to be successful it should be done, not on those already showing signs of coronary disease, but on healthy people in whom prevention would be more clearly demonstrated, (primary prevention as opposed to secondary prevention).

Cholesterol-lowering drugs

Research by ICI had meanwhile successfully evolved a drug, Clofibrate, designed to lower blood cholesterol levels; the commercial promotion of such drugs, especially in the USA, was to play a significant role in coronary prevention programmes. Nearer home, the eagerness of local consultants to prescribe Clofibrate for certain patients presented their GP with difficult decisions; it seemed to me to be as unlikely that the integrity of our hearts should depend on a new pill as on a new brand of margarine, and if cholesterol was seen as essential for normal bodily function, surely we lower it artificially at our peril? My patients were therefore free to choose for themselves whether or not the new drug should be taken; my advice given with humility was not to take it. One patient who ignored my advice and continued taking the drug for some six years was to die of cancer; I know that an isolated case like this is mere unscientific 'anecdote', but in a small practice it cannot be forgotten. Nor can the colleague who, about this time (mid 1960s), in a friendly tea-time discussion, gently chided me when I insisted that refined carbohydrates, not natural fats, were the more likely culprits in the coronary debate; I had amused him by declining his offer of exotic, highly sweetened cakes; he was sure, as he tucked into the cakes, that the evidence incriminating saturated fats was sound; shortly after our discussion he suffered a fatal coronary attack.

'Unfortunately, the patient died'

No qualms about the wisdom of using a new cholesterol-lowering drug to banish CDH were evidently felt by those who sponsored a large WHO European trial. Some ten and a half thousand men aged between 30 and 59 living in the cities of Edinburgh, Budapest and Prague were divided into two matched groups and from 1972 observed over a period of approximately 5.3 years. The first group took a daily dose of Clofibrate, the other, an inert capsule. Blood cholesterol levels fell by between 8.8 and 9.7 per cent in the drug-taking group, so in this respect the exercise was a modest success; results were published in 1978.[3]

'And what of the outcome?' wrote the author of a leading article in *The Lancet*. 'To put it briefly, "the treatment was successful but unfortunately, the patient died".'[4] *The Lancet*'s gloomy comment reflected the following disturbing results:

1. Deaths from coronary disease were the same in both groups. Lowering cholesterol had had no effect on CDH mortality.
2. In all three cities, an alarming increase (37 per cent) in deaths from causes other than CDH occurred in the first group (with lower cholesterol levels); abdominal cancer featured prominently in the range of diseases causing increased mortality.
3. A marked increase in gall stones followed the lowering of cholesterol.
4. So did a significant increase in the use of drugs for the treatment of diabetes.
5. The only benefit observed was a 26 per cent reduction in mild or non-fatal heart attacks.

Following the publication of the WHO trial, Clofibrate was immediately banned in West Germany, but no one knows whether the alarming outcome was the result of some unsuspected effect of the drug, or whether it was caused by lowering blood cholesterol.

Lesson from America

In USA in the 1950s large sums of public money had been spent on efforts to find the cause and so to prevent CDH; a sense of urgency for this research came in 1951 from the disturbing findings of post-mortem examinations on American soldiers, killed in Korea, where pathologists found signs of advanced coronary artery disease in 77 per cent of young men, aged on average 22 years; the disease evidently started at a much earlier age than had hitherto been suspected.

US research identified smoking, high blood pressure and raised blood cholesterol levels as risk factors, but large-scale attempts to reduce the risks failed, as in Europe, to bring about any improvement in overall death rates. By now, however, the cholesterol/dietary fat theory had taken such firm hold on academic circles that any dissent-

3. Committee of Principal Investigators, WHO Co-operative Trial, *British Heart Journal*, no. 40 (1978), pp. 1069–1118
4. Leading article, 'Clofibrate: A Final Verdict?', *The Lancet*, 8100, vol. 2 (1989), pp. 1131–5

ing voices, however sound their arguments, tended to be ignored or, like Dr Dedichen in Norway, censored. In the world of power politics, Solzhenitsyn coined the phrase 'the censorship of fashion' which, like the new term 'politically correct', describes the process of creeping dictatorship to which those vested with political, or in this case academic, power seem to be terribly prone. In some academic circles the urge to dominate assumes a quasi-religious quality, possibly a substitute for the traditional faith discarded by many scientists.

The 'censorship of fashion' came into its own in the USA in 1987 with the launching of the 'National Cholesterol Education Program', a colossal government-funded campaign to screen the blood cholesterol values of the entire US adult population and then vigorously to treat about a quarter of them for the rest of their lives. The programme is a warning of what can happen when a tightly knit band of highly specialised academics enjoys the official blessing of government health departments and the power to spend public money in putting their pet theory, however shaky its foundations, into practice. When this union of government and professional interest has the backing of the wealth of powerful pharmaceutical and food manufacturing empires, dissident voices have little chance of being heard.

A review of the programme by Thomas Moore,[5] entitled 'The cholesterol myth' tells of the pitfalls of the union of commercial pressures and professional arrogance:

> Although the effort appeared to be a public-service campaign, it was, in reality, a business scheme to sell products and physicians' services ... The National Cholesterol Education Programme guidelines suggested that treatment should not begin without a complete physical, and a laboratory work up ... Thus a programme that may have begun in sincere but misguided zeal for the public good became entwined with greed. The world was learning how much money could be made by scaring people about cholesterol.[6]

A new cholesterol-lowering drug, lovastatin (or Mevacor), produced by Merck Sharp and Dohme, although not yet subjected to long-term testing, was to be used in the national programme; the drug firm was thus deeply involved in the programme's promotion, especially in a campaign to change the minds of doctors unconvinced about the benefits of cholesterol-lowering by drugs or diet.

5. T. J. Moore, 'The Cholesterol Myth', *The Atlantic Monthly*, 264, no. 3 (1990), pp. 37–70
6. *Ibid.*, p. 52

The launching of the National Cholesterol Education Program is surprising in view of failure of any of the cholesterol-lowering surveys to demonstrate any improvement in overall death rates by altering dietary fats, and in view of the fact that some studies had confirmed the European WHO Clofibrate research which revealed an increase in cancer incidence associated with lower blood cholesterol levels.[7,8] We still do not know if cholesterol and associated compounds in body fluids have some protective role against cancer; nor do we know whether low blood cholesterol causes cancer, or whether cancer causes low cholesterol; commonsense would surely suggest that until we do know more, to attempt to lower cholesterol on a national scale is little short of crazy. The only benefit revealed in American cholesterol lowering campaigns is some reduction in non-fatal heart attacks; but any reduction in cardiac death rates has been invariably offset by increased deaths from other causes.[9]

Cholesterol and violence

Of these other causes, deaths from violence, accident and suicide are prominent and have now been repeatedly recorded; we must therefore ask: as well as increasing the risk of our dying of cancer, does artificially lowering serum cholesterol also drive us to violent insanity and self-destruction?

An account in *The Lancet* (1992)[10] of the role of cholesterol in brain function gives one explanation of the link between violent, anti-social behaviour and the lowering of cholesterol. A brain hormone called serotonin is known to affect human behaviour by controlling our violent impulses; cholesterol is one of the lipids (fatty complexes) on cell membranes which facilitate the transport of substances including serotonin into the brain cell. Research reveals that human subjects, including criminals with anti-social personalities, have lower blood cholesterol levels than control groups; mental hospital patients with high cholesterol are less regressed and withdrawn than those with low levels. Monkeys, fed on a diet such as now officially recommended in the USA, low in saturated fat and cholesterol, were significantly more

7. A. Schatzkin, P. R. Taylor and others, 'Serum Cholesterol and Cancer in the NHANNES I Epidemiological Follow Up Study', *The Lancet*, 8554, vol. 2 (1988), pp. 298–30
8. G. Rose, H. Blackburn, A. Keys and others, 'Colon Cancer and Blood Cholesterol', *The Lancet*, 7850, vol. 1 (1974), pp. 181–3
9. M. F. Muldoon, S. B. Manuck, K. A. Matthews, 'Lowering Cholesterol Concentrations and Mortality', *BMJ*, vol. 301 (1990), pp. 309–14
10. H. Engleberg, 'Low Serum Cholesterol and Suicide', *The Lancet*, vol. 339 (1992), pp. 727–8

aggressive than control animals on a normal diet.[11] Lower cholesterol levels, according to the author of *The Lancet* article, so alter the fluidity of brain cell membranes that the transport of serotonin is impaired; deficiency of serotonin in brain cells, in turn, weakens the natural human control of irrational violence.

American death rates

Defenders of the dietary fat theory of CDH are, I am sure, longing to remind me that in America over the last twenty years a 42 per cent fall in coronary deaths has occurred and that this proves the efficacy of the US dietary policy on cholesterol and fat consumption; but if we look at the history of CDH in America during this century we find no support at all for the belief that traditional dietary fats are the cause. From the early 1900s, as in Britain, coronary death rates in America rose to an alarming peak in 1963. From 1909 to 1961, while this sad mortality increased, a 12 per cent increase in fat consumption in America was due mostly to a rise in the supply of oils and unsaturated fats.[12] As in Norway, vegetable oils, supposed to protect us from CDH, failed to do so.

The steep decline in US coronary deaths during the 1970s and 80s started before the cholesterol lowering programme; it can best be explained by an apparently marked decline in sugar consumption, a curb on cigarette smoking, improved treatment of high blood pressure, and a massive increase in the numbers of coronary bypass operations; the reduction in per caput sugar consumption appears to have been considerable, from 47.5 kg. in 1958 to 30.2 kg. in 1987.

The Cardiff study

In Britain, the promotion of the fat theory of coronary heart disease, although smaller in scale than in the USA, had the same features; groups and committees emerged and campaigned for polyunsaturated fats, sometimes assisted by public money. Margarine vendors spent lavishly in targeting doctors with booklets, diet sheets, essay competitions and so on. The selective use of data at times verged on the farcical as even the most highly qualified scientists appeared to be ruled by ideology and fashion rather than by objectivity.

For instance, in 1991 doctors carrying out research on heart disease for the Medical Research Council at Cardiff, published their results

11. J. R. Kaplan, 'The Effect of Fat and Cholesterol and Aggressive Behaviour in Monkeys', *Psychosomatic Medicine*, vol. 52 (1990), pp. 226–7
12. M. A. Antar and others, *American Journal of Clinical Nutrition*, vol. 14 (1964), p. 169

on a ten-year study of 4000 men.[13] They found that men who drank a pint of milk daily suffered about half the number of heart attacks of those who drank no milk; they also found that men who ate butter had fewer heart attacks than those who chose polyunsaturated spreads. This finding, completely at variance with the prevailing dogma, must have brought consternation in the higher echelons on the Medical Research Council. Within a few weeks of the publication of the Cardiff study, a four-man panel of the MRC issued a statement which urged people to ignore it.[14] The panel mentioned certain defects in the design of the study, which, according to the four wise men, gave no grounds for altering the dogma that polyunsaturated fat was good, and dairy fat was bad.

Would the panel have been called and this advice issued if the results of the Cardiff study had confirmed, rather than contradicted fashionable dogma? I think not. Moreover, are not the supposed defects of the study – the use of questionnaires in assessing human diets – common to most publicly funded research projects on nutrition and health? Are we, therefore, to ignore them all? As taxpayers who contribute £200 million to the MRC, we are bound to ask why our money is being spent on long and expensive studies, the results of which we are told to ignore. If our interpretation of the outcome of research of this kind is to be dictated by a small elite of specialists, is not this a good example of the censorship of fashion and of creeping academic dictatorship?

Coronaries in the Caribbean
My support of Cleave's thesis that dietary sugar, rather than fat, caused the upsurge of coronary disease in Britain and America during this century involved me in an interesting debate with one of the most ardent and prolific champions of the virtues of polyunsaturated margarine, the late Dr Richard Turner.

In 1977 an article by Dr Turner and Mr I. S. Robertson, headlined 'Attack on Fat' appeared in the *Scottish Farmer*.[15] I was given space to reply in a later issue in which I outlined Cleave's research.[16] Later, in the correspondence columns, Dr Turner dismissed the sugar hypothesis and stated, *without giving any references or figures*, that populations in the Caribbean have the highest consumption of sugar in the

---

13. P. C. Elwood and others, *Epidemiological Studies of Cardiovascular Disease, Progress Report (1991)*, Medical Research Council Epidemiological Unit, Penarth, South Glamorgan
14. P. Pallot, Research on milk and heart attacks 'should be ignored', *Daily Telegraph*, 23 March 1991
15. I. S. Robertson and R. W. D. Turner, 'Attack on Fat', *Scottish Farmer*, 4402, vol. 85 (1977), pp. 19–20
16. W. W. Yellowlees, 'Defence of Fats', *Scottish Farmer*, 4407, vol. 85 (1977), p. 54

world, but do not suffer from coronary heart disease. My final letter in this exchange pointed out that some thirteen countries bordered the Caribbean Sea and that some of them had very low intakes of refined sugar; according to past trade figures published by FAO ending in 1958, Dr Turner's statement was not true; only in Cuba and Barbados did per caput consumption approach that of the UK. I wrote: 'If, with increased trade, these Caribbean countries are now eating sugar on a scale comparable with Britain and America, and if Cleave's theory is correct, we can predict that in an other decade or so, the unfortunate Caribbeans will begin to suffer from coronary disease as we do'.[17]

This forecast seems to have been confirmed. Exactly a decade after publication of the *Scottish Farmer* debate, the Caribbean Food and Nutrition Institute Quarterly journal, *Cajanus*, carried a series of articles on nutrition and chronic disease from which the following extracts are quoted:

Diabetes, hypertension, coronary artery disease and cancers are common, chronic, non-communicable disorders which are responsible for the majority of deaths in Caribbean countries.[18]

In almost all countries of the region, the diseases of over-nutrition (obesity, diabetes, hypertension, stroke and coronary heart disease) and malignant neoplasms are major public health problems among adults.[19]

Rats and diabetes in Dominica

Writing from the Princess Margaret Hospital in Dominica, Drs Cooles and Paul state that diabetes is an increasing problem in the West Indies and that five per cent of Dominicans are diabetic. As evidence of the seriousness of this diabetes epidemic, they report four alarming cases in which the feet of sleeping diabetics were gnawed by rats; diabetic nerve damage brought complete loss of sensation to the feet of these unhappy patients who felt nothing and were not awakened by the nocturnal attack.

If, as these reports suggest, diabetes and CDH are now common causes of death and disability in the Caribbean, the relative intake of fats and carbohydrates in that region, as shown in the table below, does not appear to favour the theory that fats are to blame.

17. W. W. Yellowlees, Letter to Editor, *Scottish Farmer*, 4412, vol. 85 (1977)
18. H. Knox, 'Nutrition and Mortality Trends in the Caribbean Region', *Cajanus*, vol. 20, no. 2 (1987), p. 87
19. Marcia H. Magnus, 'Dietary Guidelines to Reduce Cardiovascular and Cancer risk in the Caribbean' *Cajanus*, vol. 20, no. 2 (1987)

Country	Calories	Protein %	Carbohydrate %	Fat %
Barbados	3207	10	62.4	27.6
Bahamas	2422	11.6	54.9	33.4
Dominica	2109	10.8	67.9	21.3

Table 6: Daily per caput intake and percentage of calories derived from protein, carbohydrate and fat

(Source: *Cajanus*, vol. 20, no. 2, 1987)

In Britain, in order to avoid heart attacks, we are urged to reduce our fat intake to 35 per cent of total calories; the Caribbean average, well below that figure, does not appear to be beneficial. No data are given in the *Cajanus* reports to reveal the proportion of refined sugar in the carbohydrate fraction of the diet.

COMA in the wilderness

From time to time the Committee on Medical Aspects of Food Policy (COMA) appoints panels of experts to report to the government's Chief Medical Officer on subjects of special interest. The COMA panel report, 'Dietary Sugars and Human Disease', published in 1989,[20] was, of course, eagerly studied by followers of Cleave. Their surprise can be imagined when they searched in vain the awesome list of 237 references for any mention of all of the publications of the man who had done so much to elucidate the crucial role of refined sugar in the causation of twentieth-century disease.

Here is what I mean by a 'wilderness' of confusion in research on nutrition and health. I have related in chapter 7 how a group of leading medical scientists thought so highly of Cleave's contribution to our understanding of the cause and thus to the prevention of many serious diseases that they awarded him the highest accolade in the land; they bracketed his discoveries with those of Pasteur, Lister and Fleming. But here, a decade later, is another group of leading medical scientists who, on reviewing the subject of Cleave's research make no reference to him at all; and who conclude that sugar consumption plays no part in the cause of CDH.

Maybe the answer to this mystery is to be found in a revealing comment by a member of the COMA panel: 'We must not expect too much of this report. Committees are always cautious and tend to escape contentious issues by falling back on the verdict Not Proven.

20. Department of Health, *Dietary Sugars and Human Health*, No. 37 (London, HMSO, 1989)

With chronic human disease it is almost impossible to prove the cause and most dietary studies are easy to criticise on technical grounds'.[21]

If, as tax payers, we must not expect too much from such a report (at £9.80 for a slim paperback it is unlikely to be a best seller!), we have every right to ask why bother to publish it at all? Especially if such a prestigious document includes biased and inaccurate statements now to be detailed.

The Caribbean again

In dealing with sugars and cardiovascular disease the COMA panel repeats Dr Turner's assertion about sugar consumption and CDH in the Caribbean as follows: 'countries like Cuba, Venezuela, Colombia, Costa Rica and Honduras have very high consumption of sucrose and low rates of CDH'. Unlike Dr Turner, the COMA report gives two references to support this bold statement, one from the *American Journal of Clinical Nutrition* (1966),[22] the other from the journal *Atherosclerosis* (1971).[23] As I sent away to the library for photocopies of the relevant articles, I wondered: was Cleave mistaken after all? But when the articles arrived I could not help feeling astonishment mixed with mounting anger as I searched in vain for any information on either sugar consumption or mortality rates in the countries listed. In plain language, the references given in the COMA Report are bogus and according to WHO mortality statistics and the Sugar Year Book, the statement about the five Caribbean countries is false. For instance, Cuba, with the highest per caput intake of sugar in the region, has a higher death rate from myocardial infarction (i.e. coronary thrombosis) in men aged 55–64 than the USA. The discovery of such falsehoods in a document by distinguished academics chosen to advise governments is a very serious business; whom are we to believe? We have learned from the journal *Cajanus*, quoted above, how coronary thrombosis, diabetes and obesity are common diseases in the Caribbean. The 'experts' of COMA sitting in London tell us that this is not true.

Prejudice or truth

I have dwelt on the COMA Caribbean statement because it demonstrates the genesis of the wilderness of confusion on the dietary cause

---

21. K. Heaton, 'The Founders of Modern Nutrition: Cleave', (London, McCarrison Society, 1988)
22. Alfredo Lopez and others, 'Some Interesting Relationships between Dietary Carbohydrates and Serum Cholesterol', *American Journal of Clinical Nutrition*, vol. 18 (1966), pp. 149–53
23. A. Keys, 'Sucrose in the diet and coronary heart disease', *Atherosclerosis*, vol. 14 (1971), pp. 193–202

of heart disease, a wilderness created by the bias of specialists who, in pursuit of narrow dogma, seem to have abandoned the accepted disciplines of academic writing. We should also remember, when discussing national death rates in relation to a specific foodstuff like sugar, that true comparisons may be difficult in countries with poorly developed standards of medical care where accurate figures of death rates may not be available; trade figures of import and export of sugar may not always accurately reflect the per caput consumption.

I am sure that readers would wish to point out that in dwelling on the role of refined sugar I am myself assuming the 'specialist' attitude which I have been at such pains to condemn in others; they would also wish to criticise me for not referring to studies done in this country many years ago which concluded that no link existed between high sugar intake and coronary heart disease. But no dietary trials, designed to test Cleave's theories, have, as far as I know, ever been carried out in this or any other country. Such trials would have to compare, over a period of some fifty years, the incidence of CDH in two similar population groups. The study group would eat, on average, some 45 kg. per caput of sugar annually and all its other carbohydrate, i.e. wheatflour or rice, would be refined. The control group's sugar intake would be limited to the per caput ration which prevailed in Britain in the early nineteenth century, about 6 kg., and its edible grains would all be unrefined. The fact that a trial of this kind will always be impracticable gives great importance to observations, some of which I have given, of the prevalence of CDH among populations whose isolation cuts them off from access to sugar and confectioneries. No population, isolated in this way, has ever been found to suffer as we do from diabetes or CDH.

The Medical Research Council survey[24] on sugar consumption and coronary heart disease usually quoted in this context used hospital patients for its control population; some of these patients suffered from varicose veins, appendicitis or large bowel cancer, all conditions associated with high sugar consumption; there was therefore no true control group and the failure to observe any difference in rates of CDH in the control and study group is not surprising.

If I am still accused of being in the grip of my own 'narrow dogma' and of having a one-track mind on sugar I can only remind my critics of the theme of this book: human health depends above all on sound nutrition; sound nutrition means growing food and using it in accord-

---

24. MRC Report 'Dietary sugar intake in men with myocardial infarction', *The Lancet*, 7686, vol. 2 (1970), pp. 1265–71

ance with nature's laws; of all foods made 'unnatural' by industrial processing the commonest are refined sugar, refined flour and certain processed vegetable oils. I know of no research which refutes this simple concept.

22 Remembrance: Battles Long Ago

Armistice Day in Aberfeldy is often cold, grey and wet. In the years immediately following Hitler's war, the local branch of the British Legion would parade in the square and march in three ranks to the little arched war memorial nearby. In those early years, as we stood with bowed heads, it was easy to see ourselves in battle dress, manning trucks, jeeps, Bren gun carriers, guns, ambulances and tanks; to see the fields and orchards with their slit trenches, the beaches, dust and deserts of foreign lands; to hear again, against a background of gunfire, the oaths of men and officers, the shouted commands, and in spite of the hell of it all, the jokes or even laughter.

But as the years and then the decades have come and gone, our numbers have dwindled; memories of war have faded. The formal parade has been abandoned; we are now a small cluster of elderly, grey-haired men and women, standing round the memorial while the Sunday traffic passes down the main street, uncaring even in the two minutes' silence.

The voice of the minister comes fitfully through the noise of the traffic and the whisper of wind, gusting in the trees: 'Age shall not weary them, nor the years condemn. At the going down of the sun and in the morning, we will remember them'.

Year by year, I make a special effort to remember them, especially my brother Robin, who in 1940 left his farm in Argyll to join the RAF; like him, so many whom I knew went cheerfully, and like him, many of those with most to give did not come back.

The interlude of war which took my generation to foreign lands and untold hardships greatly affected our later attitudes and created a huge gap between us and the rising generation. Compared with the horrors of World War I what many of us endured on active service in Europe was, I suppose, a mere picnic; but even without the unspeakable terror and degradation of prolonged trench warfare, death and wounds and mortal danger are stern teachers which bring new dimensions to human thought. When we returned to civilian life, many of us felt the sad contrast between the sense of common purpose, sacrifice and comradeship of the war years with the decline, in the post-war decades, of so many aspects of our national life.

The October 1936 intake of medical students, of which I was one, were fortunate; by September 1939, when Neville Chamberlain told us that we were at war with Germany, we had passed our second professional examination and were strongly advised, in the national interest, to continue our studies. So, while many of our contemporaries, like both my brothers, left their chosen careers to join up and to face the anguish of defeat and disaster in the first two years of war, we medical students remained in our lecture theatres and laboratories in the tranquillity of wartime Edinburgh, an Edinburgh as yet unspoilt by post-war traffic and by the awful ugliness of modern architecture, where lumbering trams took you anywhere in the city for a few pence and the shopper could park his or her car in Princes Street.

By the spring of 1942, having completed the statutory six months' post-graduate resident hospital job, we were ready to exchange our junior hospital doctor's white coat for a medical officer's uniform. I thought it unfair that a medical degree should immediately confer the status of first lieutenant, a rank only achieved by combatants after arduous training. At Glasgow's Central Station, as I boarded the train to take me to the RAMC training depot at Leeds, I was embarrassed to receive a respectful salute from a young second lieutenant who, as we journeyed, told me of the severity of his training. When he asked me where I had been, I had to confess only to a well-known gents' outfitters where in exchange for my uniform allowance my uniform had been fitted and supplied.

As a doctor in uniform, I never quite succeeded in dispelling the sense of being an imposter among real warriors who had been schooled to endure the rigours of battle; three weeks' training at the RAMC Depot did little to prepare young doctors for the reality of war. The field ambulance to which I was posted, under the command of an alcoholic colonel – by 11 a.m. daily he was usually drunk – accentuated feelings of unreality, disillusionment and boredom.

Suddenly, however, in the autumn of 1942, we found ourselves in a troop train bound for Greenock on the Clyde estuary. Talk and rumour of the opening of a second front had for months been rife. This, it seemed, was it. Whither were we bound – another Salonika, France, Greece, Egypt?

The ships of every description which crammed the estuary off Greenock gradually made for open sea. Out in the grey Atlantic the immense size of our convoy convinced us of the importance of our mission; ahead and astern of our liner (the P&O *Strathnaver*) were ship upon ship, as far as the eye could see. On each flank, like busy sheepdogs guarding their flocks, destroyers threw up white bow waves as they plunged and weaved through Atlantic rollers.

After a few days voyaging south, sealed orders having been opened, all was revealed. Our armada, a joint British-American force, was to land on the North and West African coasts and to secure ports in Morocco, Algeria and Tunisia; these would supply General Anderson's First Army as it pressed eastward to seize the main bases of Rommel's Afrika Korps at Tunis and Bizerta. The operation, code-named Torch, under the command of an American general called Eisenhower, sought to free the Mediterranean from enemy control and to prepare the way for attack on southern Europe. As we arrived off the North African coast, we heard over the ship's radio that at El Alamein Montgomery's Eighth Army had won a famous victory, and that the German Afrika Korps was already in full retreat.

Having paused in the bay of Algiers for some forty-eight hours, our ship, with supporting vessels, sailed east in darkness to the small port of Bougie where, as we anchored at dawn, the relative comfort of our voyage so far was rudely shattered. Enemy aircraft were now reacting vigorously; one of the larger ships of our convoy, already hit by bombs, listed and burned. The *Strathnaver*'s Oerlikon anti-aircraft guns blazed away as we climbed down scramble nets to the landing craft which delivered us safely to the docks; I was ordered to open a first-aid post to deal with casualties and sickness among the dock-operating companies.

German and Italian bombers came over, sometimes by day, but mostly by night to dive-bomb the docks; they were greeted with an increasingly impressive barrage and, although casualties remained surprisingly light, ships were hit and set on fire. Dive-bombing had a personal terror; the steady drone of a formation of propellor-driven planes gives way to the crescendo of the dive, then comes the whine of falling bombs, each one of which seems to be aimed at oneself. Before my first-aid squad had time to dig shelters, we slept, when sleep was possible, in a flimsy dockside warehouse alongside heaps of dried figs, ready for packing and export; we enjoyed eating the occasional fig, but did not relish the sound of anti-aircraft shrapnel splintering the tiles.

Within days, experience confirmed what had been taught in RAMC training, that in war, casualties from wounds are always outnumbered by those from sickness. By day, our post dealt with increasing numbers of diarrhoeas, skin rashes, coughs and so on, by night with the bombers. We had certainly ceased to be bored; but endured some unpleasant nights as we struggled to rescue casualties from burning ships.

After some three weeks at Bougie, orders arrived for us to move inland by train. Wartime shortages of coal had forced the Algerian railway to eke out fuel for its steam engines with dried wild briar roots. Piles of roots dotted the verges of the track which meandered through the majestic valleys of the Atlas mountains.

The First Army had failed in its dash to reach Tunis and Bizerta in the weeks after landing and was to be held in bitter fighting during the winter months in the mountains overlooking the plain of Tunis. As a corps field ambulance, our tasks during the winter were not heavy. We listened eagerly to radio reports of Montgomery's Eighth Army as it fought and pursued the German Afrika Corps for 1800 miles from Egypt to the Tunisian border.

On 5 May 1943, the First Army, reinforced by the Eighth, launched a final attack from the mountain pass at Megez el Bab, broke the German line and thirty-six hours later was in Tunis; 248,000 prisoners were taken.

In the throng of soldiers, prisoners, and refugees which now milled about Tunis and its suburbs, the sand-coloured vehicles of the Eighth Army mingled with our First Army green camouflage; for the first time I saw the HD signs of the 51st Highland Division and with joy greeted various friends. In a few weeks the posting to the Highland Division which I had asked for came through and took me to the 175 Highland Field Ambulance at the port of Sousse; there, with assorted landing craft, 152 Brigade with its Field Ambulance prepared for the invasion of another unknown shore.

With great relief we set sail on 8 July; a hot wind, the sirocco, coming off the Sahara like a blast from an oven had made life in Sousse extremely unpleasant. We passed by Malta and learned that we were bound for Sicily. Off the Sicilian coast, at Cap Passero, landing craft unloading on the beach and various ships at anchor remained unmolested from air, land or sea; as far as we were concerned the operation was unopposed and soon our 152 Brigade vehicles pressed inland through villages, farms and vineyards.

On 13 July the brigade met stiff opposition at a hill village called Franconfonte from units of the 2nd German Paratroop Regiment. Casualties, some severe, from Seaforth and Cameron Highlanders began arriving at our Advance Dressing Station; on the 14th, the Cameron Commanding Officer, Colonel Sorel-Cameron, and his medical officer, Captain Montgomery, both wounded by the same mortar bomb, were among the new casualties. I was asked to pack my kit and to report immediately to the Camerons as the replacement Medical Officer. 'Doctor,' Colonel Cameron shouted to me from his stretcher, as I left our small reception tent, 'watch out as you go, for snipers in the orange groves.'

I couldn't help reflecting what an easy target I was for even a cockeyed sniper, as I sat with the driver, perched in the front seat of the large Austin ambulance given for the journey! We drove past brigade HQ vehicles drawn up at the side of the road, then past a battery of 25-pounder guns shelling a target across the valley, then along a stretch of road threateningly empty of all movement, with orange trees on either side. We got lost, but at last came on Cameron HQ and a small group of men and officers crouching beside an anti-tank gun. A large, cheerful, moustached man greeted me, shook me warmly by the hand and said how glad they were to see me; he was the battalion padre, the Reverend Coty Smith, a man whom I came to admire and revere. He chatted as if I had arrived at his manse for tea and I tried not to notice the crackle of machine-gun fire among the trees as he introduced me to the adjutant and to my sergeant and stretcher bearers. The padre assured me that although the machine gun making all the noise was a German Spandau, it had been captured by the Camerons and was not now firing in our direction!

In thus becoming a regimental medical officer, I quickly learned the truth of the paradox that in the army, the nearer you get to the sharp end, the more likely you are to encounter a spirit of friendship, cheerfulness, sardonic humour and a sense of purpose, attitudes in marked contrast to those prevailing in some units enjoying the easier life of the base areas. I came to admire the professional skill of battalion NCOs and officers, not only in the use of their weapons, but in the way they led and nurtured their men.

The family embrace given by the regiment to all those who come under its wing could be sensed by a newcomer even in the chaos of this Sicilian skirmish, which had seen the sudden removal of the commanding officer and responsibility for the conduct of the battle entrusted to Major Noble.

In his concern for the welfare of men and officers the inspiring influence of Padre Smith was a powerful force in maintaining morale. He seemed to know no fear; far beyond the call of his duties, he would go out with stretcher bearers, out with night patrols; his presence gave strength to the weak, courage to the fearful, of whom there can have been few more fearful than the new medical officer! There was no forced cheerfulness nor bravado in his Christian humility. The officers and men of the 5th Battalion were maybe not famed for their piety, but they turned up willingly to his services, held in the field. They worshipped this cheerful saint. The faith which I now have owes much to the example of Coty Smith; if he embodied the Christian church in action, here was an example to be followed.

Who would true valour see, let him come hither;
One here will constant be, come wind, come weather.

In the terrible wilderness of war, thanks to men such as this, virtue not only survives, but shines all the brighter. As I wrote these words on this June day of 1992, by a strange telepathic coincidence the phone rang; it was Colonel Tom Lamb, distinguished ex-adjutant of 5th Camerons, calling to tell me that he had just attended the funeral of Coty Smith who, by then in his eighties, had died. The trumpets must have sounded with a special note of triumph for this good and faithful servant.

Only those who have experienced war can know what is expected of the men and officers in an infantry battalion: in the face of danger, endurance beyond human limits, marching, digging, fighting, by day and by night, fatigue to the point of tears, blessed relief to be able to sleep briefly in a grubby slit trench. All this demanded a very high standard of fitness; but by 1943 new recruits to infantry units were not always up to A1 standards. It was said that after the fittest and most able men had joined commandos or paratroops, Britain was 'scraping the barrel' to replenish the ranks of its infantry battalions.

But the spirit of the Highland Division embodied in its commander, Major-General Douglas Wimberley, moulded unpromising human material into a formidable fighting force. The General's lanky figure bestrode the battle field and heartened his men; his uniform often seemed ill-fitting, but his dedication to the tactical task of the day dominated his every movement and his manner was sometimes more like that of a keen professor who was going to solve the problem ahead in the best way possible. Faith in his ability and his enthusiasm somehow seemed to percolate down to the humblest foot soldier. Another source of strength in Highland regiments lay in the close bond between officers, NCOs and men, a bond often based on shared territorial roots with maybe a lingering trace of clan kinship.

Long practice had brought to near perfection the cooperation of infantry and supporting 25-pounder artillery regiments. We were soon to hold, for a few days, a God-forsaken position by Sferro railway station overlooked by our foes, established in the surrounding hills. The least movement by day was greeted by a shower of mortar bombs. Our security held good, thanks, it seemed, to the skill and coolness of our attached artillery forward observation officer who, for ever gazing through his binoculars as he leaned against a wall, answered the mortars with well-directed artillery fire and gave his radioed instructions to the guns away behind us, as if he was ordering groceries.

Sferro Hills

The enemy had checked our advance in the hope of stopping us from encircling the port of Catania with its airfields; the strong point of their line of defence in the Sferro Hills, flanking the plain of Catania, would have to be taken if our movement was to continue. This required a set-piece attack and was my first and most vivid experience of what was to be repeated many times in the following two years as the Division launched attack after attack on its way, via Normandy, through France, Holland and Germany.

In his briefing of the Divisional officers round a sand-table model of the Sferro Hills, the General gave his usual masterful résumé of what was required in the coming attack; to a novice in this world of infantry movement his grasp of detail of the how and when was deeply impressive, especially his comprehensive account of the location and extent of the German defences dug in on the hill. The attack, to be led by 152 Brigade, would be by night, initiated by a massive artillery barrage. On the day before the attack we would have to lie up concealed behind the ridge on our side of the valley we were to cross.

The shallow dip on the hillside gave no shade at all from the pitiless blaze of the July sun; we had marched there during the night but could not now sleep because of the heat; a few shells came over, but none very close. With nightfall we moved in single file over the ridge and down a goat track to the floor of the valley; the track had been marked with shaded lamps and white tape, but on the flat the indicators seemed to give out and we got lost as we groped our way over the dry river-bed to the start line. For a while all was total confusion, as the time for the barrage fast approached; at last with much whispered cursing we got sorted out on the line, companies in front.

I lay for a moment on my back and gazed at the heavens; the dim outline of the low hills could just be seen against the stars; I had never seen so many of them against such a black velvet sky:

> When I consider the heavens, the work of thy fingers, the moon and the stars which thou hast ordained;
> What is man that thou art mindful of him. . . .

How infinitely insignificant our creeping about on this arid island in the face of the immensity of the universe; what has the Creator in his mind as He beholds the follies of His creature? As I lay there I remembered lying exhausted on the grass of an Argyll glen, after gathering sheep on my brother's farm, dozing to the soothing noise of water running over waterfalls. Here there was no water, only heat and dust; the silence of the night was broken by the faint rustling of movement of the waiting battalion, the clink of boot metal on stone, whispered instructions.

Suddenly, blinding flashes danced and blazed in the sky behind us, a split second's pause before the deafening thunder of the barrage shattered the night; then the air above us was full of the silken whine and rush of shells. Some three hundred yards ahead the earth erupted in a long line of orange-coloured flame, grey dust and smoke; instinctively one pressed one's body against the earth; from the thudding of exploding shells it seemed as if a thousand terrible horsemen were galloping up the valley floor.

Soon the line of fire and smoke moved forward; we followed walking slowly. No need for silence now in this hellish din as we shouted to keep together; was there a kind of terrible ecstasy as we walked to the tune of the guns? Two parallel lines of red tracer shells, fired overhead by Bofors anti-aircraft guns, gave us the correct line of advance. We started to climb as the barrage lifted to the higher slopes where lay the main part of the enemy defence system. Surely nothing could live in that awful concentration of shell fire. As if in answer to such a thought, the rip and crackle of Spandau machine-guns sent silver streaks of tracers whistling and fizzing around us as we stopped in a little wadi; the crump of hand-grenades and the rip of small-arms fire now added to the din as we began to receive and collect the walking wounded, including some German, ashen faced, trembling. All enmity seemed lost between those united in the pain of their wounds and the terror they had endured. To examine, assess and dress those wounds in the semi-darkness was not easy; flares dropped from a plane (theirs or ours?) gave intermittent light.

The hectic business of cutting away uniforms to expose sometimes hideous wounds, the problem of how best to treat or splint mercifully banish all sense of fear and horror; a job has to be done and to be immersed in the job is to forget everything else. At first light, when I went to battalion HQ and managed to get a couple of jeeps to take wounded back, I heard that our blokes had taken the hilltop objective but a counter-attack with tanks was now in progress. Quite a few shells were coming our way, among them, according to the experts, armour-piercing shells from the counter-attacking tanks. 'Cup of tea, sir?'; oh, blessed relief! The brewing of tea comes high on the priority of therapies. The MO's staff could brew tea under any circumstance. Tea and a cigarette were sometimes as potent as morphine in calming a trembling, wounded soldier. Tea – relief not only from the tea itself, but because it stood for normality and for the humanity which might somehow survive this present hell. The counter-attack failed; three tanks were knocked out by our anti-tank guns, but still wounded came.

As the new day advanced and the noise and dust had settled, the Brigadier, Gordon MacMillan, arrived at our battalion HQ to tell us that all objectives had been taken and the battle appeared to be won. In the relative quiet we could at last snatch some sleep, then try and assess losses in dead and wounded. We had lost five officers and forty other ranks killed or wounded. The bodies of some sixty German and Italian soldiers were to be buried on the hill.

That was the virtual end of German resistance in Sicily; elsewhere on the island, Canadians and Americans were rapidly closing on Messina. From the Sferro hilltop we could gaze on the vista of green vineyards, olive groves and woods on the lower slopes of Mount Etna.

So in Sicily, for a while, one apocalyptic horseman – Conquest and War – had been locked up; but in his place had come the pale horse of Pestilence. Padre Smith lay fevered and shivering in his slit trench, refusing to be evacuated to hospital; the malaria which had laid him low now incapacitated scores of officers and men, who filled base hospitals. An epidemic of jaundice added to the toll of casualties far greater in number than those of battle.

My reverie by the war memorial was broken by the piper playing 'The Flowers of the Forest' that haunting tune which evokes, down the centuries, the infinite anguish and sadness of the loss of Scotland's young manhood.

In quiet corners of far-flung continents and islands neat rows of headstones mark their sacrifice.

Lord God of Hosts be with us yet
Lest we forget—lest we forget.

The Flowers of the Forest. Real flowers graced that ancient forest of pine, birch, rowan and oak; its carpet of grasses and shrubs teemed with life. But just as man's inhumanity to man caused countless thousands to die in war, so man's ignorance and folly has cleared all but a few tiny remnants of the old trees from Scotlands mountains and glens. No flowers bloom beneath the blanket of closely packed conifers now being massively planted on bare slopes; no life flourishes underneath those rows of alien trees.

23 Remembrance: Decline and Fall

If the men who perished in the service of this country in Europe, North Africa, the Middle East, Burma and on other far continents and oceans were to return today, as from a long journey, I wonder what their feelings would be. Those who fell in 1940 as Hitler's panzers raced to the channel, when the conquest of our islands seemed only a matter of time, would be relieved to know that we are not after all a province of the Third Reich.

We have been spared the horror of the dictator state – secret police, imprisonment and torture, the knock on the door in the small hours, the terror, spying and all-pervading fear. We remain free within the law and can still express our opinions without the risk of being carted off to perish in some ghastly gulag. In this respect those whom we remember would surely be glad that they had not died in vain. They would be glad, also, to see a dwindling of class differences and an increase in material wealth undreamed of in pre-war years.

They might, however, be dismayed to learn what we are doing with the freedom for which they gave their lives. What would they think of the tragic decline in standards of truth and morality, the destruction of the family, increasing robbery and violence, the assaults and murders, the fear of elderly people in some of our cities to walk out after dark? Has the loss of so many fine men in two world wars depleted our national store of wise leadership and hastened the process of decline and disintegration?

Doomed civilisations
It is a fitting postscript to last chapter's thoughts on Armistice Day to quote the words of a distinguished and wise soldier, the late Sir John

Glubb, who spent much of his service career in the lands which gave birth to European civilisation:

> Long periods of wealth and power corrupted these nations; money became more important to them, replacing the old standards of honour. Their wealthy descendants, living in luxury, saw less need for Divine aid. Religion became a sheer formality, sexual morality was abandoned and money assumed paramount importance. Crimes of violence became everyday events. The leaders ceased to be statesmen and became politicians, bribing, lying and intriguing in pursuit of their private interests. The exact repetition of the signs of decline in empire after empire over thousands of years is amazing. Such peculiarities, for example, were the public infatuation for athletes, actors, and singers which is recorded of the Greek empire, Rome, Byzantium and the Bagdad of the Kaliphs.[1]

The only difference between that picture of the decline of ancient civilisations and what is happening in Britain today is that radio, television and new communication techniques have given added power to those who wish to pursue their private interests by 'intriguing and lying'.

To the generation of white-haired veterans standing by the war memorial the changes in morals and behaviour since World War II are a constant source of amazement. Crimes of violence have indeed become 'everyday events'; child abuse, rape, adultery, perversion, murder, robbery seem to occur on an unprecedented scale and to be the only theme in the minds of those who write and produce plays for television. Marriage is derided as an outmoded institution; church membership continues to dwindle.

In deploring these trends, are we merely expressing, as the elderly always have done, the sour thoughts of crabbed old age? I think not; changes as profound as these do not come about by chance; they come through the deliberate and sometimes carefully planned actions of influential people. Radio and television have played a crucial role in an onslaught on the Christian religion. It is, of course, an onslaught which began on that first Easter when the crowd, gathered outside the palace of Pontius Pilate, shouted for the release of Barabbas, not Jesus. Crowds are seldom swayed thus without the instigation of

---

1. Sir J. B. Glubb, *The Way of Love* (London, Hodder and Stoughton, 1974)

power-hungry leaders, 'lying and cheating in pursuit of private interests'; they shouted for the release of a convicted terrorist, not for the Saviour of the world.

Permissive society

In modern times certain scientists, particularly social scientists, caught up in ideologies heavily laced with Marx and Freud, have been in the forefront of the attack on Christianity, which they have seen as an outmoded superstition standing in the way of human progress and of individual freedom. In the UK and elsewhere the coming of the permissive society marked the triumph of this new ideology.

An early inkling of the arrival of the permissive society came in 1962, in the choice of that year's BBC Reith lecturer,[2] the late Professor Carstairs. Here was a distinguished psychiatrist inferring, in the third lecture, that 'sexual experience with precautions against conception is becoming a sensible preliminary to marriage, a preliminary which makes it more likely that marriage when it comes will be a mutually considerate and mutually satisfying partnership'. This all sounded so civilised, so relaxed, so sure that old-fashioned beliefs on the desirability of chastity should be swept away in order to usher in a new age of human 'satisfaction'.

In earlier chapters of this book I have suggested that in the field of prevention, academic specialists are not always wise counsellors; examples of how they will distort evidence in order to further their particular theory were given in chapter 21. Here are two further examples of this process from the Reith Lecture briefly quoted from above:

1. As a model for the joys of the permissive age, the Reith lecturer referred to sociological studies of various tribes including the Samoans.[3] But according to press reports of later research, done by an American university team, the Samoans, far from being gentle people, have about the highest rates of rape and murder in the world; the original sociological studies in Samoa referred to by the lecturer were seriously flawed.

2. 'Sexual experience with precautions against conception is becoming a sensible preliminary to marriage': this bold assertion does not take into account that many adolescents, as is known to any GP, go through a period of utter gormlessness which renders them quite incapable of taking 'precautions against conception'. In Sweden com-

2. M. Carstairs, *This Island Now* (London, Hogarth Press, 1962)
3. M. Mead, *Coming of Age in Samoa* (London, Penguin Books, 1943)

pulsory sex education for children over ten, which started in the early 1950s, was followed, in the 1960s, by a marked rise in illegitimate births, abortions and sexually transmitted diseases, especially in the fifteen- to nineteen-year-old age groups.[4]

In reviewing *Sex and Society in Sweden*, a book which detailed these changes in sexual habits,[5] a psychiatrist, well known in his day, wrote:

> It is surprising to learn that the incidence of syphilis and gonorrhoea is steadily increasing in Sweden and especially in the fifteen to nineteen age groups. There are parallel increases in illegitimate births and requests for abortion.
>
> Some sort of devil must be at work here, wrecking the good and persistent efforts of several generations of honest people who tried their best to clear society from hypocrisy and narrow minded prejudice and to create in their place a world of self respecting freedom and equality.

Do you really clear society of 'hypocrisy and narrow-minded prejudice' by forcing ten-year-old children into sex education classes? The AIDS virus has, of course, arrived since this review was written in 1969; the Devil (not just 'some devil') is having a great time!

In the two decades following 1960 the sad harvest reaped from permissiveness in the UK is similar to that in Sweden; the proportion of conceptions ending in abortion has risen from 7 per cent in 1969 to 20 per cent in 1988. Record figures for divorce, illegitimate births, sexually transmitted diseases and child abuse hardly support the theory that in the new permissive climate marriage becomes more 'mutually considerate and mutually satisfying'. A report, published in June 1992 by the Office of Population Censuses and Surveys finds that 'the marriages of those who live together before marriage were 60 per cent more likely to end in breakdown'.

Precocious puberty

One of the most remarkable biological happenings in the last one hundred and fifty years is the fall in the age of onset of puberty in girls from seventeen, early in the 19th century, to thirteen and a half in modern times (it is now nearer eleven or twelve). In mentioning this phenomenon, the Reith lecturer gave as its cause improved health

---

4. B. Linner, *Sex and Society in Sweden* (London, Jonathan Cape, 1968)
5. M. Balint, review of *Sex and Society in Sweden* by B. Linner and R. Litell, *BMJ*, 5656, vol. 2 (1969), p. 564

and nutrition. In a long review of the falling age of puberty, Tanner revealed similar trends in Scandinavia, Germany, Britain and the USA.[6] In these countries, in 1810, maximum stature was not achieved until twenty-five years of age: now it is reached at eighteen to nineteen in males and sixteen to seventeen in females. Tanner's studies suggest that this tendency to earlier maturation (and presumably to earlier sexual activity) started in Europe and America in about 1840. The nutritional cause of earlier maturation is thought by some biologists to be increased consumption of high quality protein.

But we saw in chapter 15 how recent research in Europe, America and the Canadian Arctic linked the lowering of the age of puberty and acceleration in growth rate in adolescents not with increased protein consumption, but with mounting intake of refined sugar. 1840, the year which, according to Tanner, marked the start of the growth spurt, was also the year when, with the removal of import duties, a steep rise started in Britain in the manufacture and consumption of refined sugar. These studies repeat the fascinating question posed in Chapter 21 in my review of the results of artificially lowering cholesterol levels: can human behaviour be influenced by food quality as well as by custom, law or religion?

The question is not far-fetched. In McCarrison's classic rat-feeding experiments, rats fed on the standard control diet of whole grain cereals with fresh butter, fresh fruits, vegetables and milk ad lib, lived happily together; those on a 'poor class British diet' featuring white bread, margarine, tinned jam, tinned meat, over-cooked vegetables and much sweetened tea were nervous and apt to bite the attendants: stronger rats began to kill and eat the weaker ones of the group and had to be segregated.[7] We have already seen how eating refined sugar leads via hyperinsulinism to disharmony of the human hormone orchestra of which sex hormones are important instruments. Are modern teenagers, their hormones thus unbalanced, in the grip of precocious sex drives which are not matched or checked by adult mental maturity?

Here is another wilderness of ignorance; but before we get too carried away by the effects of unnatural foods on human behaviour, we should remember that Cain slew his brother Abel before refined sugar, cholesterol, white bread or margarine were thought of.

---

6. J. M. Tanner, *Education and Physical Growth* (University of London Press, 1961)
7. R. McCarrison, *Nutrition and Health* (London, Faber, 1953), pp. 29–30

The family

Whatever the effects of processed, unnatural foods on human behaviour, there is no doubt of the success of those who established the permissive society by waging war on Christianity and by bringing about the wholesale destruction of the family.

As the cell is the unit of living tissues in plants, animals and human beings so the family is the biological unit of human (and many animal) communities. When cells disintegrate, living tissues cease properly to function and the whole organism becomes ill. So do disintegrating families bring about disintegrating communities. In Britain over one third of marriages now break up; by 1988 some 25 per cent of children under sixteen experienced the divorce of their parents[8] and will themselves have increased difficulty in making stable adult relationships. Thus about one quarter of the coming generation is likely to be handicapped in maintaining the integrity of their families.

If the good seeds of education, obedience, respect for law are not sown in the family, a harvest is reaped of chaos in schools, falling educational standards and rising crime rates, the sad hallmarks of the 'post-Christian' society. In our colleges and universities during the last two centuries many scientists, philosophers and intellectuals have laboured to bring about this state of affairs; they worship not at the shrine of a living God, but in temples of scientific advancement. Science has blessed us with near-miraculous benefits which can lift from the human lot much misery, suffering and disease; but if advancement in science is not matched by reverence for creation, misery and chaos are apt to replace any hope of human contentment. The following extract is from a paper, 'All the World's a Stage', read at a conference on psychiatry in general practice, held by the Royal College of General Practitioners:[9]

On the stage of Christendom, in seeking guidance to those profound problems of personal and national life . . . the people traditionally put at the centre of their stage, the man of God, the preacher in his pulpit. Even if both preacher and audience failed hopelessly down the centuries to live up to the message that was preached, nonetheless, in all walks of life formal recognition was given to an optimistic divine purpose and to the active presence of the Devil. But over the last two hundred years the audience has become increasingly bored

8. W. Oddie, 'Repairing a generation of damage to the family', *Daily Telegraph*, 22 November 1990
9. W. W. Yellowlees, 'All the world's a stage', *Journal of the Royal College of General Practitioners*, 17, no. 82, supplement No. 3 (1969)

with this kind of sermon, and the reason for their distraction has been the dramatic entry of a flamboyant character, the Wizard. In the dramatis personae of this fantasia the Wizard is described as: 'a technocrat or technologist who believes in human salvation through scientific and industrial advancement; despises the preacher'.

The Wizard's performance has been impressive and he deserves the thunderous applause he has been given as act follows act, moon rockets and monoamine oxidase inhibitors, atomic fission and television, jet propulsion and juke boxes, computers and contraceptive pills; no wonder that the preacher has forgotten his words; but the Wizard has become so pleased with himself – he knows not the meaning of the word humility, and is a chap of endless conceit – that he has pushed the preacher into the wings, put on his robes, mounted the pulpit and started preaching sermons . . . Now a pulpit is no place for a Wizard, and his elevation there is a dangerous thing, dangerous because his sermon is based on the rather nebulous Freudian doctrine that the chief end of man is the pursuit of personal wealth and pleasure and touches not at all on the inescapable knowledge of good and evil . . . If we are to look forward to a society which has stability and purpose, and therefore mental health, we must seriously think of putting the Wizard in his place before the curtain is run down in chaos and darkness.

24 Remembrance: Land and People

In his account of the decline of ancient empires of the Middle East, Sir John Glubb omitted one feature of imperial decline, widely agreed by historians: the dwindling of the power and influence of Babylon, Greece, Carthage and Rome followed the erosion of their soils, erosion brought about by overcropping, deforestation, extractive farming and rural depopulation. The dissipation of human energies in war hastened the process.[1] The decline of spiritual values detailed by Sir John seems to have gone hand in hand with the loss of soil fertility.

Soil degradation

Again we have to ask the question about the quality of food and human behaviour: does loss of soil fertility so affect quality as to impair human energies and abilities? We shall never know the answer to that question, but we do know that throughout human history destruction and degradation of soils have followed unwise extractive farming. A dramatic example occurred in the North American Middle West in the 1890s; monoculture, the use of modern machinery and chemical fertilisers in the course of some thirty-five years turned into dust and desert a vast territory of virgin fertile soil. In the two decades between 1914 and 1934 the world lost more fertile soil than at any other time in human history.[2]

Farmers of past civilisations, and even those who created the American dust bowl, could be forgiven because of their ignorance. Today we have no such excuse.

---

1. Edward Hyams, *Soil and Civilisation* (London, John Murray, 1976), p. 115
2. G. V. Jacks and R. O. White, *The Rape of the Earth* (London, Faber, 1949)

'Organic' dawn

The late Sir Albert Howard, a pioneering champion of biological or 'organic' farming, demonstrated in the 1930s the crucial role of **living** soil organisms, bacteria, fungi, worms etc., in the growth of healthy crops; after extensive research on the beneficial effects of composts on soil fertility and studies on the health of stock reared on biologically grown fodder, he concluded that most agricultural research, done by chemists and specialists on small plots, was obsolete and irrelevant.[3]

Howard's work inspired Lady Eve Balfour to launch the Haughley experiment in Suffolk in 1939 – the first attempt ever to compare, *on a farm scale*, organic and chemical methods, by measuring, as far as possible, yields and quality of crops and stock. In 1935 another ecological venture, the Peckham experiment,[4] conceived by Dr Scott-Williamson and Dr Innes Pearce, sought to study the health of 2000 families whose social and recreational activities were centered in a new purpose-built building in Peckham in London. The interest aroused by the publication of *The Peckham Experiment* in 1943 and a few months later by the appearance of Lady Eve's book, *The Living Soil*[5], brought the authors together; with other like-minded scientists and farmers they founded the Soil Association, a body which thus sprang from a union of medicine and agriculture. In 1947 the newly fledged Soil Association took over the running and financing of the Haughley experiment.

In her book, Lady Eve listed the pioneers whose writings had inspired her: they included Sir Robert McCarrison, Weston Price, Francis Pottinger Jnr. and Sir Albert Howard. Of them she wrote:

These pioneers have one thing in common – they were what we should now call ecologists. They all succeeded in breaking away from the narrow confines of the preconceived ideas that dominated the scientific thinking of their day. They looked at the living world from a new perspective – they also asked new questions. Instead of the contemporary obsessions with disease and its causes, they set out to discover the causes of health. This lead inevitably to an awareness of wholeness (the two words, after all, have the same origin) and to a gradual understanding that all life is one.

3. A. Howard, *An Agricultural Testament* (London, Faber, 1950)
4. I. H. Pearce and L. H. Crocker, *The Peckham Experiment* (London, Allen and Unwin, 1943)
5. Lady Eve Balfour, *The Living Soil* (London, Faber, 1943)
6. R. McCarrison, *Nutrition and National Health* (London, Faber, 1944)

The first objective of the new association, 'to bring together all those working for a fuller understanding of the vital relationships between soil, plant, animal and man', challenged the orthodoxy of the time. Here was an ecological approach which put prevention at the forefront of medicine and agriculture. In founding the Soil Association Lady Eve Balfour had taken Sir Robert McCarrison as her chief mentor.

McCarrison's Cantor Lectures, delivered in 1936, appeared in a slim hard back, *Nutrition and National Health*, published by Faber in 1944. In Faber's second edition published in 1953, in order to avoid confusion with publications about the newly established National Health Service, the title was shortened to *Nutrition and Health*. After McCarrison's death in 1960 the late Dr Hugh Sinclair, one of his staunch admirers, took charge of Sir Robert's research papers and wrote a postscript for a third edition by Faber in 1961. In 1982 Faber relinquished the copyright of the book to enable the McCarrison Society to publish a fourth edition.

The Medical Testament

McCarrison's teaching had deeply influenced an energetic general practitioner, the late Dr Lionel Picton, secretary of the Cheshire Local Medical and Panel Committee representing 600 general practitioners. In 1938, led by Dr Picton, the Cheshire Committee issued its famous Medical Testament[7] which pointed out that since the inception of the National Health Insurance Act of 1911, while death rates had fallen, the incidence of ill-health had greatly increased; in this respect the act had been a failure (the same unfortunate outcome holds for the NHS Act of 1948). The Cheshire Medical Testament, which quoted extensively from McCarrison's research, ended with the following statement:

> We are not specialists, nor scientists, nor agriculturists. We represent the family doctors of a great county ... We cannot do more than point out the means of health ... We are called upon to cure sickness. We conceive it to be our duty in the present state of knowledge to point out that much, perhaps most, of this sickness is preventable and would be prevented by the right feeding of our people.

Triumph of chemists

The publication of the Cheshire Medical Testament, the Peckham

---

7. L. J. Picton, *Thoughts on Feeding* (London, Faber, 1946), p. 22

experiment, the founding of the Soil Association, and the writings of Howard and McCarrison appeared to be setting the scene after World War II for health promotion through a union of medical and agricultural research. But in the years that followed, no such union took place; rather, fragmentation in the biological sciences continued; medical schools, uninterested in prevention, concentrated on highly specialised studies of disease; an ecological approach to nutrition and health played little part in their curriculae and the advocacy of health-giving food was seen as the raving of cranks. When, in 1968, I approached the chairman of the education committee of the Royal College of General Practitioners and asked for a conference featuring nutrition and health, I could sense, in his response, the alarm, almost the horror, at such a proposal! That serious general practitioners should concern themselves with such things as wholemeal bread and fresh vegetables to him was absurd.

In the three decades following the end of World War II for all but a small minority of the population white bread remained the bread of choice and the consumption of refined sugar greatly increased. In 1973 lack of funds and policy disagreements brought the Haughley experiment to an untimely end just as important results were beginning to emerge. On most farms in the UK the input of soluble chemicals and new pesticides increased enormously; advocates of organic methods were derided as 'muck and mystery' idiots, while academic research in medicine remained completely divorced from research in agriculture.

Mycorrhizal association

These trends bring us back to the controversy between science and religion. Soil fertility depends on living energies, living relationships in the top few inches of the soil. The most important of these is mycorrhizal association – the fascinating partnership between certain soil fungi and the root hairs of many plants. By penetrating the substance of root hairs these fungi enable the plant to absorb essential nutrients, and, according to the work of Howard, to resist disease. Here is one of nature's miraculous living partnerships.

Where there is life there must be reverence; the organic grower tries to revere and to emulate nature's laws and processes by encouraging mycorrhizal association and by seeking to enhance soil fertility for future generations. This he does by using natural wastes to build up the humus content of the soil and to feed the soil's living population.

The chemist, the 'wizard in the pulpit', has no reverence for living systems, his chemicals depress mycorrhizal association and unnaturally boost plant growth at the expense of disease resistance; a battery of toxic pesticides is called on to protect the plant. Loss of humus brings soil erosion; leached soluble nitrates pollute water supplies; the chemical system runs at an energy loss and in the long term cannot be sustained. Possibly the worst feature of orthodox chemical agriculture is its addictive quality; to maintain harvests from new high-yielding seed varieties, more and more artificial chemicals are required;[8] and because natural fertility is depressed by chemicals, the farmer who wishes to convert to organic or biological methods has to face several years' greatly reduced yields.

My garden plot

A retired GP, who is not faced with the daunting task of making a living as a farmer in the chaotic conditions of the European Community's Common Agricultural Policy, is maybe in no position to pontificate on farming; but the crisis which now faces our agriculture – farmers being paid not to farm – is surely the culmination of a long history of academic and government policies which ignore the unique place of land use as the basis of human health. Official policies for farming, as in so many other spheres, have been heavily influenced by urban-based industrial interests; thus agriculture is geared not to conserve the health of our soils for future generations, but simply to sell chemicals.

In previous chapters I have told of my attempts to discover if good garden crops could be grown on soil fertilised only by composts and without the use of any soluble fertilisers or toxic pesticides; to illustrate the success of this exercise in organic growing even in the hostile environment of an exposed, stone-covered hillside, I have listed crops available for eating in the hungry months of April and May, the months of scarcity before summer's harvests are available.

Autumn-sown vegetables

Some overwintered under cloches.
1. Lettuces (Winter Density). 2. Spring onions (White Lisbon).
3. Spinach beet (Swiss chard). 4. Purple sprouting broccoli.
5. Spring cabbage. 6. Various herbs.

---

8. C. Gopalan, 'Nutrition and Growth', Proceedings of the Royal College of Physicians of Edinburgh, vol. 22 (1992), p. 166

Stored crops harvested last autumn

Stored in straw or peat in wooden bins kept in the garage. 1. Potatoes.
I have continued to use my own seed potatoes for some forty years.
2. Carrots. 3. Parsnips. 4. Beetroot. 5. Jerusalem artichokes. Main crop
onions store well in bunches hanging in the shelter of the porch. Leeks,
one of the most versatile of all garden crops, remain in the ground;
but in mid-winter a pickaxe is sometimes necessary to lift them from
hard frozen ground, so we take the precaution of shoving ('sheughing')
a supply in the soil of the greenhouse.

Organic gardening is not trouble free; the usual pests and diseases
are encountered, but losses are seldom on a scale which seriously
affects overall yields and there does seem to be a vigour in growth
which makes unnecessary recourse to toxic pesticides.

An organic example

In 1985 Ian Millar of Jamesfield farm in Fife became convinced that
with the ever-increasing use of chemical fertilisers, the soil of his 300-
acre farm was degrading; he wanted to hand on to future generations
land that was in good heart and so decided that he must change
course and build up real fertility by organic methods. He now harvests
a variety of vegetables for sale to retailers, lettuce, cabbage, carrot,
broccoli, potatoes; and also grows cereals, wheat, barley and oats. He
hopes to enlarge a small herd of cattle to make a better balance
between stock and crops.

He and his wife do not regret their decision; they have the satisfaction of seeing the fertility of their fields improve year after year;
partridges and other wild life which had been declining are now
flourishing. One of their greatest difficulties was in knowing how best
to go about the conversion from chemical to biological farming, since
no official authority evidently is equipped to advise the farmer who
wishes to go organic. The addictive nature of chemicals causes a
dramatic fall in yields for possibly five years until the soil regains its
natural fertility. Having got over this critical phase, cereal yields at
Jamesfield are now comparable to those grown with chemicals.

Successful organic farms refute the claim, so often made by spokesmen of the orthodox school, that a heavy input of chemicals is absolutely necessary in modern agriculture. These farms give a golden
opportunity for the college academics to come down from their ivory
towers, to come away from their small-plot experiments and to study
whole-farm systems with a view to improving soil fertility by biologi-

cal methods; they may be surprised by what they find in this unfamiliar world. For instance, Mr Millar has confirmed that thanks to a rising population of earth worms soil pH remains stable and liming is not required. There is tremendous scope for research on non-chemical methods of weed control and on the various methods of enhancing and maintaining the life of the soil. At Jamesfield new implements like the Brush Weeder and the Tearaway 2000 are proving highly effective substitutes for herbicides.

It is unlikely, however, that new machines can obviate the need for a return of farm workers to the empty cottages which have not already been taken over by holidaymakers. Organic farming holds out the hope of reversing the relentless drain of skilled workers from the land; some 9000 farm workers departed from Scottish farms between 1980 and 1990.[9] Surely this loss is to be deplored, especially at a time when the destination of these skilled workers may well be the dole queue.

I do not know how widespread in Scotland is the disquiet on official fertiliser policy, expressed in the following extract from a letter from a Dumfriesshire stock-rearing farmer:

Unfortunately a situation has been allowed to develop in which advisers and researchers have come to believe in the infallibility of their experimentation and scientific knowledge, with the consequence that they are failing properly to address a wide range of pressing practical problems, such as:
Soil structure deterioration and under-liming;
manganese deficiency in grass and cereals;
hypomagnesaemia and molybdenosis in cattle;
the broken-mouthed condition in ewes.

My experience indicates that the cause of each of these problems is closely linked with the use of ammonium nitrate in the manner recommended by the Scottish colleges of agriculture and that their fertiliser recommendations have never been properly tested or evaluated.[10]

Trace element deficiency
Another farmer, a dairyman in south-west Scotland who in 1976 accepted official advice which seemed not to have been 'properly evaluated and tested', experienced widespread trouble in his dairy

9. R. Crabtree, Z. Appleton and others, *The Economics of Countryside Access in Scotland* (Aberdeen, Scottish Agricultural College, 1992)
10. T. Stockdale, Woodcroft farm, Dumfriesshire, personal communication, 1989

herd especially at calving time.[11] He had participated in an EEC-based scheme designed to boost the output of dairy farmers and so to bring their income up to the levels of pay or salary enjoyed by workers and managers in industry. The official advice under the scheme was to double the number of milking cows on his 180 acres and to use intensively nitrogenous fertilisers featuring a heavy input of ammonium nitrate. The serious and widespread sickness which then appeared in the enlarged herd was found to be associated with selenium deficiency. His cows and calves were restored to health by the use of selenium supplements given in special capsules. Other milk producers whose cows graze south-west Scotland's lush pastures and who participated in the new regime have experienced serious trouble from copper deficiency.

In discussing the cause of the prevalence of cancer in Scotland (chapter 10), I mentioned a possible association of cancer incidence with deficiency of certain trace elements in crops fertilised intensively by the use of chemicals. Since I wrote that chapter, reports of research in Finland state that minorities of the population having low levels of selenium in their bodies had over three times greater risk of getting cancer.[12] Studies in many countries have shown that animals with selenium deficiency have a greater risk of suffering from cancer.[13]

Selenium is obviously an essential protective element; like some vitamins, in large doses it can be toxic; amounts of selenium in the soil vary throughout the world; they are lower in lands overlying igneous rocks as in parts of Scotland, in Scandinavia and in New Zealand.[14] Crops grown by intensive chemical application, especially in those regions, tend to have dangerously low selenium levels, which leads to widespread sickness in animals.

For reasons stated in my introduction, scientific proof of trace element deficiency as a cause of human cancer, brought about by the intensive use of soluble chemicals, will **always** elude us. If, in such a vital matter, science cannot help us, if we cannot ever know certainties, we can only fall back on human intuition which would surely urge caution, and question the ever-mounting load of artificial chemicals put on farm lands. Caution is equally called for in the use of modern pesticides.

---

11. J. Scott Park, Portnellan Farm, Gartocharn, personal communication, 1989
12. Arthur Wynn, 'Selenium: Do We Need More?' McCarrison Society Newsletter, spring 1990, p. 11
13. *Ibid*
14. *Ibid*

Pesticide Peril

In 1963 the publication of Rachael Carson's book, *Silent Spring*,[15] set alarm bells ringing which even the most bigoted scientist could not ignore. In language easily understood by the ordinary reader, *Silent Spring* gives a who's who of the modern herbicides and pesticides, most of which, being manmade, occur nowhere in nature and are therefore not biodegradable. These toxic substances have a devastating capacity to disrupt and destroy the basic systems of life; some can enter human bodies by skin contact; the chlorinated hydrocarbons, of which DDT and dieldrin are examples, persist indefinitely in the tissues of man, beasts, fish and birds.

Organophosphates

The organophosphates (OPs), derived from chemical warfare 'nerve gases', include sarin, malathion, parathion, mipafox and others. They are less persistent than the DDT group and are supposed to be less toxic than the original nerve gas; OPs are widely used as pesticides in farm and garden. Recent studies in America have shown that long-term exposure to low doses causes measurable disturbance of brain function.[16] Exposure to larger doses causes tremors, mental breakdown, convulsions and death.

Small quantities of modern pesticides are now regularly detected in human blood and mothers' milk. In new departments of environmental medicine, increasing numbers of patients are being seen whose immune systems show measurable signs of breakdown as a result of this chemical onslaught.[17] The annual incidence of accidental poisoning of humans, animals and fish, sometimes on a horrendous scale, from spillage of these poisons and their spread in the food chain to even the remotest corners of the earth, would surely argue for a complete and immediate ban on their use.

Pesticides: cancer in America and Britain

Studies in the USA have shown that between the early 1950s and the 1970s differences in cancer occurrence between rural and urban populations have tended to disappear. The lower rates of cancer deaths

15. Rachael Carson, *Silent Spring* (London, Hamish Hamilton, 1962)
16. F. H. Duff and others, 'Long-term effects of organophosphates on human encephalogram', *Toxicology and Applied Pharmicology*, vol. 147 (1979), pp. 161–79
17. W. J. Rae and Liang Hsueh-chia, *The Effects of Pesticides on the Immune System* (Environmental Medicine Foundation, Breakspear Hospital, Abbotts Langley, Herts, seminar of 14 October, 1989)

traditionally noted in rural areas no longer hold.[18] During the same period, the 1950s – the 1970s, the use of herbicides and insecticides has greatly increased. The dose of herbicide used in corn growing rose from 70.5 million pounds of active ingredient in 1964 to 420.4 million pounds in 1982. Herbicide use was strongly associated with genital and lymphatic cancer.[19] The authors of this study urge caution in interpreting results and call for more research in a possible link between agricultural chemical use and cancer mortality. Other studies in America confirm the upsurge of cancer in rural areas. 'The cancer rate in the nearly industry-free farming state of Iowa is about the same as the number one cancer-producing chemical dump state of New Jersey'.[20]

The drift of toxic chemical sprays is now a problem on a global scale. Pesticides against grasshoppers, sprayed in central Africa, were detected five days later in Florida in the United States; they were then traced as they followed the Gulf Stream up the east coast of America to Bermuda, thence off towards Europe.[21]

The enormous scale of the use of pesticides in Britain is suggested in one estimate that in 1983 well over one thousand million gallons of pesticide-carrying spray was showered on to farming land.[22] According to a report of the British Pesticides Action network, data from the Office of Population Censuses and Surveys reveal higher rates of congenital malformations in the children of agricultural workers, gardeners and groundsmen than in the offspring of workers in other occupations.[23] Again, in reviewing these findings, we cannot be sure of cause and effect; exact measurements, as I have emphasised throughout this book, are impossible. We have to guess and in doing so to use our commonsense and our capacity for wise decisions. We can, however, dismiss as nonsense the assurances of spokesmen for the chemical industry who state that, if used according to instructions, modern pesticides are perfectly safe. In America, where methods of analysis seem to be more advanced than in this country, virtually 100 per cent of the food supply contains traces of herbicides and pesticides.[24]

18. Shannon Stokes and Kathy Brace, 'Agricultural Chemical Use and Cancer Mortality in Selected Rural Counties in USA', *Journal of Rural Studies*, 4, no. 3 (1988), pp. 239–47
19. *Ibid.*, p. 245
20. W. J. Rae and Liang Hsueh-chia, *The Effects of Pesticides on the Immune System* (1989)
21. *Ibid*
22. Jean Munro, 'What Agribusiness Does to You', *Soil Association Journal*, September 1984
23. *Ibid*
24. W. J. Rae and Liang Hsueh-chia, *The Effects of pesticides on the Immune System* (1989)

A Doctor in the Wilderness

Pesticides in the Third World

If, in the industrial West, danger from pesticides lies mostly in long-term exposure to low-level contamination of food and environment, recent estimates published by the WHO seem to show that in the Third World the perils of acute serious poisoning are near catastrophic. One estimate puts the annual number of severe acute poisonings at three million, with 220,000 deaths. The same source estimates that 25 million agricultural workers annually suffer a minor poisoning episode.[25] In Sri Lanka in 1982, out of a population of 12 million there were 1000 deaths from acute pesticide poisoning.[26] Many of the episodes of acute serious poisoning, possibly two thirds, are suicides, especially from the use of paraquat; evidently this herbicide, now so easily accessible, is a major means of suicide in the Third World.

None of us knows if the health-giving quality of biologically grown food is due to non-toxic levels of nitrate, to the absence of pesticide residues, to higher levels of vitamins, to a correct balance of minerals and trace elements, to some other unknown quality or to a combination of all of these; but I am sure that those consumers who are prepared to spend time and money in obtaining organic produce are acting wisely.

Thanks to the continuing work of the Soil Association and the Henry Doubleday Research Association (see Appendix I), interest in organic farming and gardening is steadily growing. The demand for organically grown food has exceeded supply, a trend which, in time of recession, may be checked because of the higher prices charged by organic growers.

Since first working on this chapter, I have visited the garden at Auchterhouse, near Dundee, tended by Mr Cameron Thomson and his wife. They are convinced of the urgent need to re-mineralise the earth's soils by the use of appropriate rock dust and hope to establish a Scottish earth regeneration trust. Their garden, fertilised by rock dust fortified by goat dung litter, certainly is good evidence of the success of their beliefs.

25. *The Lancet*, Noticeboard, 'Pesticides in the Third World', 8278, vol. 336 (1990), p. 1437
26. *Ibid*

25   Hell on Earth

In preceding chapters I have dwelt on two main reasons for the wilderness of confusion over the dietary cause of many of the serious diseases prevalent today. They are the frailty of human nature on the part of scientists, engaged in nutrition research, who get hold of an idea and refuse to accept any evidence, however compelling, which casts doubt on its veracity; and, secondly, the dominant role of commercial interests in determining the dietary habits of consumers, as well as in shaping developments in agriculture and in medical practice.

I cannot avoid linking both reasons with a decline, in recent history, of spiritual values and the retreat of Christianity. Doctors are repeatedly told that on no account must they be 'judgemental', nor must they 'moralise'. But doctors are meant to be scientists and science is supposed to reveal the truths of the material world. Are doctors to remain silent when they believe that truth is being perverted?

Cheap food

As the Industrial Revolution progressed in the nineteenth century, material values triumphed over spiritual. Our leaders decided that we British should be fed by exporting goods, manufactured in our new expanding industries, in exchange for cheap imported food. The cheap food policy helped to keep industrial prices competitive, but it signalled the destruction of home agriculture as the bulwark of health through sound nutrition.

Massive rural depopulation, widespread unemployment and a cancerous growth of cities with their teeming slums resulted in a terrible imbalance between city and country and brought us to the brink of defeat by blockade and starvation in two world wars. The failure to preserve our farmlands as the main source of our sustenance and health marked a departure from wisdom; the promise of industrial wealth led to a decline in reverence for our own soil and for human dignity.

As the philosophy of the chemist and the factory conveyer belt increasingly dominated food production and farming, the imbalance of population between city and countryside increased and, in my opinion, is now the cause of human degradation on a massive scale. These thoughts do not deplore industrial efficiency and market forces as the best means of increasing material wealth by trade. When Jesus drove the traders from the precincts of the temple, He did so not because they were trading; the reason for His divine wrath was that firstly, they were trading in a place of worship, and secondly, they were trading fraudulently.

Industrial philosophy

The Christian ethic does not condemn the creation of wealth by hard work and honest trading, but as human beings work the soil and use its harvests, they are dealing not with inert material but with living forces. Where there is life there must, as in God's temple, be reverence; obedience to natural law must take precedence over the rules of the market place. Here are two examples of the consequences of applying industrial philosophy to living systems:

1. *Mad cows*. The commercial reward of converting carcase wastes, including sheep offal, into high protein feed for livestock seems an obvious way of increasing the efficiency of an abbatoir business. But the guts of sheep which carry the infective agent of Bovine Spongiform Encephalopathy (BSE) are not the natural food for herbivores; the weekly slaughter of thousands of cows, struck down by 'mad cow disease', is the price we are paying for this defiance of natural law. We cannot be absolutely sure (although it seems unlikely) that human beings will not also catch this disease.

2. *Fluoride and dental decay*. Manufacturing industries, like abbatoirs, are bound to seek a commercial outlet for as much of their wastes as possible. In North America, before the introduction of artificial fluoridation of water supplies, hydroflurosilicic acid, a highly corrosive and poisonous industrial waste product was neutralised and then thrown away. But in the 1950s the growing demand for fluoride by municipal water authorities in the US and Canada changed all that.

Here was a vast market for a product which hitherto, because of its extreme toxicity, was difficult and costly to dispose of; the use of small quantities in herbicides or rat poisons gave little scope for expanding trade. In Toronto,[1] fluorosilicic acid, a waste or by-product of the phosphate and other industries, produced at 3–4 dollars per ton, was soon to sell at 45 dollars per ton. Storage tanks used in fluoride manufacture had to be protected by special rubber linings without which this corrosive chemical would eat through the metal in a few hours.

By 1966, the Electric Reduction Coy. of Canada Ltd. was able to turn out 60 tons of the acid every day to supply the 7000 tons or more required to fluoridate ten big cities in the US. No wonder that writers of the trade journals of the time were enthusiastic about the outlook for expansion and hoped that state laws would make fluoridation of water supplies mandatory everywhere.

Hydrofluorosilicic acid is not a natural constituent of drinking water; naturally occurring fluoride in hard water from deep boreholes, ionised with calcium and magnesium, is drunk by only a tiny minority of the British population.[2] It is far less soluble and less toxic than fluorosilicic acid.[3] Moreover, the effects on human beings of ingesting the latter over a life time remain unknown.

All power corrupts

Some ten years ago, in Edinburgh's Court of Session, a lady pensioner sought to restrain Strathclyde Regional Council from fluoridating the regional water supplies. In 1983, after a very long hearing, the judge granted an interdict in the lady's favour on the grounds that to use water supplies as a means of mass medication was illegal.[4] This judgement should have brought to an end fluoridation in Scotland and the UK. (No other European country this side of what was once the Iron Curtain, apart from Ireland and the UK, now uses fluoridation.)

But the government, using the 'payroll' system of voting to ensure a majority, hastily introduced a bill to legalise fluoridation. Maybe this curious action, in a year when parliamentary time was said to be scarce, was motivated by the deep concern of our MPs for the health of children's teeth; would the Fluoridation Bill have been given such

1. A.-L. Gotzsche, *The Fluoride Question* (London, Davis-Poynter, 1975), pp. 117–8 and 135
2. Royal College of Physicians, *Fluoride, Teeth and Health* (1976)
3. G. Waldbott, *Fluoride the Great Dilemma* (Lawrence, Coronado Press Inc., 1978), p. 103
4. Opinion of Lord Jauncey, Court of session, Edinburgh (1983)

priority without the influence wielded by those whose prime concern is the health of the chemical industry?

We can well understand the enthusiasm of industrialists in north America and Britain for ever more fluoridation. It is, however, very difficult to fathom the attitude of doctors, particularly the members of a committee of the Royal College of Physicians of London whose 1976 report strongly recommended compulsory mass medication.[5]

Any doctor who, having studied the relevant research papers, advocates forced medication by fluoridation of water is either a fool or a knave; he or she defies the basic rules of medical ethics, that all patients must be treated as individuals and a doctor must never risk avoidable harm to his or her patient. Mass medication doses young and old, frail and hearty, with no regard at all for their individual make-up nor for the accuracy of dose. The possibility of harm from fluoridation is very real; many scientists, including senior dentists, have pointed to dangers;[6] others have concluded that fluoride in water does not prevent dental decay, but merely delays its onset by a few years.[7] The report of the Royal College of Physicians on fluoridation is a classic example of wilderness-creation by 'experts', who refuse to accept any evidence, however strong, which undermines their own beliefs, who are not above publishing downright falsehoods and who are prepared in their arrogance to force medicine down the throats of the entire population.

The USSR experiment

When Lenin seized power in Russian in 1917 the dictatorship of political 'scientists' and materialists triumphed over traditional beliefs in a divine purpose as revealed in the teachings of the Christian church. At the heart of all the arguments of the day on political and economic theory lay the fact that the Russian Revolution was a spiritual struggle. At last man, endowed with full control over the material world, could order affairs according to human rationality and to the teachings of Karl Marx and other political theorists; in this huge country, with its long Christian tradition, there was now no need, according to the Bolsheviks, for God nor for the inhibitions of outmoded religious beliefs. Churches were closed or destroyed; 'free love' and secular marriage were encouraged, abortion became a usual

5. Royal College of Physicians, *Fluoride, Teeth and Health* (1976)
6. P. R. N. Sutton, 'Fluoridation 1979' Submission to Committee of Inquiry, University of Melbourne (1980)
7. R. Weaver, 'The Inhibition of Dental Caries by Fluorine', Proceedings of the Royal Society of Medicine, 1973, vol. 41 (February 1948), pp. 284–90

means of birth control and believers were killed or persecuted. Farmers and peasants were deprived of their land and herded into collectives. Those who resisted, millions of them, were starved to death or butchered. The wider slaughter, torture and imprisonment without trial is now well documented.[8]

Pollution and disease. Seventy years on, with the coming of 'glasnost' and the collapse of communism in the Soviet Union and its east European empire, the world can ponder on the economic and social results of the experiment started by Lenin.

Poland, the country which in 1939 we hoped to save from Nazi dictatorship, 'has been reduced by four decades of communism to the most poisoned and polluted country in Europe. More than a third of Poland's population, 12 million people, now live in areas designated "ecological disaster zones". 70 per cent of Poland's rivers are now so toxic that they are unusable for any purpose'.[9]

In permanently smog-shrouded areas of Silesia, by the age of ten some two thirds of children suffer from serious physical and mental disabilities.[10] According to the Polish Academy of Sciences, cases of leukaemia in children have doubled within a decade: and 100 million trees have been destroyed.[11] Similar accounts from reliable sources in Czechoslovakia tell of premature human death, pollution of the environment and destruction of trees.[12]

In the Soviet Union the scale of environmental disaster is far greater, almost beyond belief: in huge inland seas, once teeming with fish, all life has been killed; and the Aral sea itself, one of the largest inland lakes in the world, is almost totally destroyed. A tenth of the habitable land area of the largest country in the world is reduced to desert.[13]

Disaster areas. In February 1992 a UNICEF/WHO mission investigated the health of the newly independent Central Asian Republics. Their report confirms that these republics are indeed disaster areas; the mission 'encountered widespread public concern about the harm done to the environment by industrial and agricultural pollution'. The report includes the following findings:

    1.   Widespread poverty and malnutrition. Vegetables, milk, fruit

---

8. A. Solzhenitsyn, *The Mortal Danger* (London, Bodley Head, 1980)
9. C. Booker, 'The East's silent sickness', *Daily Telegraph*, 17 June 1989
10. *Ibid*
11. N. Greg, 'East Europe, legacy of death', *Sunday Telegraph*, 17 June 1990
12. *Ibid*
13. C. Booker, *Daily Telegraph*, 17 June 1989

and meat are beyond the reach of most families, who have to live on bread and potatoes.

2. By our standards a very high infant mortality, 40–50 per 1000 live births. (England 9.1, Japan 4.8.)
3. Nutritional anaemia among half to three quarters of mothers. Maternal mortality is high.
4. A rising incidence of congenital disease and occupational illness and a perceived increase in cancer.[14]

Polluted land and water, diseased and malnourished mothers and children on a massive scale – to call this Hell on earth is surely not exaggerating.

Kitchen gardens for health

Death and disease on such a scale in former Soviet republics does not result from a lack of doctors. Medical services are provided free of charge with two general practitioners per 1000 population backed by an army of *feldshers* (medical assistants), nurses and midwives. About 90 per cent of this malnourished population possess television sets. It would be hard to find a better example of what happens when land use ceases to be linked to the needs of human health. Readers will be interested to know that one of the recommendations of the UNICEF/WHO mission is to 'encourage home food production through kitchen gardening'.

Here is support for my belief that, in the prevention of degenerative disease, kitchen gardens or their equivalent in land use, cultivated for fresh, organically grown food, are more important than medical services. I have described the achievements of another notable advocate of kitchen gardens for health, Dr Halley Stott, who, in setting up his clinic for malnourished Zulus in Natal, gave high priority to the demonstration organic vegetable garden.

Can it happen here?

In the West, thanks to a relative freedom from the shackles of state ownership with its corruption, inefficiency and bureaucracy, we have suffered no serious food shortages; but the rising incidence of cancer in rural areas of the USA, reported in chapter 24, is maybe a warning to affluent countries, where pollution by agrichemicals has reached unprecedented levels. It seems that, in the capitalist West, we too may

14. L. C. Chen, J. E. Rohde and R. Jolly, 'A looming crisis: Health in the Central Asian Republics', *The Lancet*, no. 339 (1992), pp. 1465–7

be in urgent need of 'kitchen gardens' and that my toil at the compost heap is perhaps not so daft after all.

Pollution and cancer

In the last two decades falling incidence of cancer of the lung and stomach in most advanced countries has been offset by an overall increase in cancer of other organs.[15] How much of this is due to contamination of food and environment by the ever-mounting load of chemical fertilisers and pesticides? We will never know, but do we not know enough to call a halt to chemical farming, especially in Scotland where, although we do not suffer frank malnutrition from hunger, congenital deformities and cancer occur more frequently than in other advanced countries?

State control or private ownership?

How can agriculture preserve the integrity of the soil, promote human health and give the farmer a good return for his toil? Not, it would seem from the result of the Soviet experiment, by state ownership of land and state control of day-to-day production; that way gives short-ages, pollution, crippling taxation and waste. In Western Europe, where land remains largely in individual ownership, food shortage seems to be a thing of the past; but the European Common Agricul-tural Policy spends enormous sums of taxpayers' money to pay for huge surpluses, for waste and for the millions lost by fraud.[16] Here are uncomfortable hints of a Soviet-style set-up. Are European 'Com-missioners' not rather similar to Soviet 'Commissars'? Some features of the late Communist empire – the concentration of agricultural production in ever-larger units and centralised control by a mush-rooming bureaucracy – have come upon us, not by the brute force of murdering armies or secret police but by the more subtle duplicity of spineless politicians, who seem uncaring as control of all our affairs are handed over to faceless European officials.

Should, therefore, all state subsidies be abolished and farm pro-duction be left entirely to market forces and to consumer demand? I do not know, but am sure that if agricultural policy is to give absolute priority to the maintenance of soil fertility and to the promotion of human health, the only possible way forward is conversion to organic or biological methods.

15. D. L. Davis, D. Hoel, and others, 'International trends in cancer mortality in France, W. Germany, Italy, Japan, England and Wales, and the USA', *The Lancet*, no. 336 (1990), pp. 474–81
16. B. Johnston, 'EC Errors have Cost Taxpayers Millions', *Daily Telegraph*, 24 October 1992

Is it not extraordinary that at a time when millions of pounds of public money are being spent in paying farmers not to produce and in storing food surpluses, no serious thought has apparently been given to use a fraction of these huge sums to keep the land in production by a programme of conversion to organic growing, where lower yields would reduce unwanted surpluses? Farming income and policy are now so completely controlled by the state that the change would have to be partially state funded; in appendix 2 I have ventured to suggest how this change might be assisted. I am well aware that my suggestions will be seen as impossible or wildly impracticable; I am no economist and I dare say they are, but somehow our policy for food production must change course.

There might be difficulty in recruiting the work-force required for labour-intensive organic farms. After several generations of city dwelling, would large enough numbers of men or women be willing to face the change to a rural setting? Are those who dwell in cities so conditioned that even the prospect of secure jobs far from busy streets holds no attraction? Why not at least explore the organic option by trying it out in a regional pilot scheme?

Failure so far to treat seriously the organic option and the very simple rules for health through sound nutrition is due, as I have suggested throughout this book, partly to the power wielded by money, a power which for ever distorts truth and before which politicians seem to be helpless. The surest defence against such power is enlightened public opinion and the ability of those who produce and sell food to meet the demands of consumers.

Consumer groups

Perhaps the best way forward for the growing number of citizens who seek organically grown food is in the formation of consumer groups who would then buy a share in an organic holding. Shareholders give the farmer security by paying him an annual salary; in return they enjoy a year-round supply of vegetables and other organically produced foodstuffs. Groups of this kind, formed by people concerned about the quality of chemically grown fruits and vegetables, are established in the USA and Japan; the shared interest of group members in their farm or market garden gives to them a warm social dimension and helps to ensure success of these valuable projects. Now similar groups are springing up in the UK.[17]

---

17. S. Dibb, 'From Farm to Your Front Door', *The Food Magazine*, 18, vol. 2 (1992), p. 6

Money power

I implore any reader who doubts the reality of the power of money in moulding dietary habits to study the final chapter of Professor John Yudkin's book *Pure, White and Deadly*.[18] Professor Yudkin held the chair of Nutrition and Dietetics at the University of London from 1954 to 1971. Researches there which convinced him of the harmful effects of the huge quantities of sugar consumed in the UK were repeatedly published in scientific journals and his views were well known. His account of the efforts of the sugar trade to silence him would be almost funny were they not so sinister: conferences at which he was to speak cancelled, censorship of his papers, character assassination so serious as to require successful legal action. If this is the way the food industry fights its battles, what hope is there for truth?

The wilderness of confusion in the minds of ordinary people about the basis of human health might be less dense if doctors paid more attention to these matters and if they understood that, as I have tried to show earlier, the cause of modern disease is, in broad outline, very simple. The recommendations given to individuals in Appendix I are essentially simple, but will probably be derided by most of my professional colleagues.

No doubt they would wish my severed head to be served up on a plate; that was the fate of the original voice in the wilderness.

---

18. J. Yudkin, *Pure, White and Deadly* (London, Penguin Books, 1986)

Epilogue

Until the day of retiring approaches, many general practitioners and, I dare say, lawyers, ministers, teachers and their helpers may not realise the strength of the bonds which, through the years, have tied them to the lives of many families. Suffering humanity leans on the shoulder of the doctor whom it knows; but, in a subtle way, the doctor becomes dependent on those who need him. For general practitioners these bonds are probably stronger in isolated rural practices. The web of family relationships, spun out of a multitude of shared anxieties and emergencies, can be a wearisome burden when at all hours the strident phone keeps ringing; but what happens to the departing doctor's ego when the phone ceases to ring and he or she is no longer needed? For fear of this unknown void, I kept postponing the decision to retire.

For many, the prospect of endless hours of the ecstasy (and agony) of the golf course banishes any risk of this dilemma; for the golfer or fisherman retiring can't come soon enough. For me the problem was solved by the potter's wheel with which, as I was nearing sixty, I had been playing in our Breadalbane Academy weekly evening art class. In the sessions taken by the academy art master and sculptor, David Rhind, I became increasingly fascinated by the miraculous transformation when a lump of spinning clay rises as a useful and perhaps beautiful vessel at the touch of the potter's hands. Here was a world of clays, glazes, firing techniques, embracing geology, history, archaeology, chemistry, physics and design. It is, of course, impossible for an aging brain to do more than skim this awesome list of subjects and they are of no use to a potter until he has fully mastered the craft of throwing. This I tried to do by attending pottery courses run by Nigel Gow and Joe Finch in Scotland, Carol Lodder in England and, in Wales, by Phillip Cunningham and Phil Rogers. All were splendid teachers and good companions.

Epilogue

My wife and I fortunately still owned a small annexe of the surgery buildings which we converted into a potter's workshop. Its windows looked on the doctors' car park. Now, as I sat at my wheel, I would sometimes see one of my former partners emerge hurriedly and drive off to some emergency. My reaction lacked any thought of envy; I felt only relief that it was no longer I who had to face a crisis of blood and tears, and that now my weighty decisions related not to human lives but to this piece of clay. But other stresses did arise; I would have to sell enough pots to cover the fearsome overheads incurred even by a hobby potter; and when in 1988 I began to write this book, the conflict between making pots and writing brought back a hint of former stresses – no time to do what I wanted to do. Are we so made that we cannot help repeating life's pattern over and over again?

I am certainly no Trollope, able to rise at 5.30 a.m. and write a thousand words per hour before breakfast; as 1992 dawned, it became painfully obvious that if ever my book was to be finished I would have to cease potting altogether. That was a painful decision, coming just as I seemed to have mastered the technique of throwing large storage jars which sell so well; this is why it has taken me almost five years to finish *A Doctor in the Wilderness*. During those years none of the developments in nutrition research makes me want to alter what I have written. I remain convinced that unless a new organic approach is brought to bear on the growing and processing of food, the burdens of ill-health, human misery, pain and economic cost will not diminish.

In the tilling of the soil and the preparation of its harvests the needs of human health and the preservation for future generations of the fertility of unpolluted land must take precedence over all other economic considerations. It is good to know that increasing numbers of consumers share this view. Here the signs are hopeful.

However, as another year ends we seem to face an ever steepening decline in our national and international affairs; lawlessness, cruelty, corruption and violence at home are matched by spreading chaos, war and famine abroad. The apocalyptic horsemen gallop all over the globe, and statesmen seem unable to stop them. Perhaps I am over-pessimistic; in the television age, are we merely seeing things as they always have been? This may be true of foreign wars and revolutions, but I am sure that the spread of lawlessness and immorality at home is real and tragic and has happened since, as a nation, we have abandoned our Christian faith. By declaring that only a return to that faith will bring us out of the wilderness, I know that in the prevailing climate of thought I will not win many friends. But I will still be in good company.

> He either fears his fate too much
> Or his deserts are small
> That dares not put it to the touch
> To gain or lose it all.[1]

Aberfeldy, January 1993

James Graham, Marquis of Montrose 'I'll never love thee more', circa 1650

APPENDIX 1

Advice to consumers

In the following two appendixes I venture to advise action by individuals and by government. I hope that appendix I will encourage readers to eat food which has the following qualities: freshness, variety, minimum amount of cooking, wholeness and the absolute minimum of artificial additives. Choose organic food if the price is affordable; the Soil Association Organic symbol guarantees against deception. The greater the consumer demand for organic produce, the more it will become available.

One sure way of getting fresh, organically grown vegetables, is to have a kitchen garden and to explore the organic way of growing. Membership of the Henry Doubleday Research Association (HDRA) (see below) is an invaluable help to organic gardeners who wish to know the delight of being able to stroll into the garden to find all the ingredients of the day's salad.

If, having changed your diet to obey these precepts, you suffer from symptoms of indigestion, or 'rheumatism', you are strongly advised to try food combining as described in chapter 2.

The following three foods should whenever possible be avoided: refined sugar, refined white flour and highly processed vegetable oils.

1. Refined sugar. Table sugar, i.e. sugar used for sweetening tea, coffee or desserts, should be cut out altogether. This is not as difficult as it sounds. The sweetening of tea or coffee is a habit akin to addiction; most people who stop taking sugar in this way for two or three weeks will find that, instead of satisfying, the sweet taste becomes repugnant. For countering the sour taste of rhubarb, gooseberries or other fruits, use natural sweeteners such as dates, raisins or figs. If for some tastes these have to be assisted by a dash of refined sugar, brown sugar sold

207

as 'Barbados' brand does contain traces of minerals and vitamins; but all sugars white and brown should be avoided as much as possible.

Probably more than half of the refined sugar being eaten in this country today comes as a food additive for a vast number of popular processed foods. These are not only sweetened drinks, sweet biscuits, sweets, ice cream, chocolate, cakes and canned fruits. Also on the list of artificially sweetened products to be avoided are canned vegetables, soups, some stews, canned baby foods and sweetened yoghurts.

Between-meal snacks featuring sweetened biscuits are a potent source of sugar; Cleave has demonstrated how such snacks contribute to the cause of acid-type dyspepsia and duodenal ulcer.[1] A cup of tea or coffee is a welcome break in morning or afternoon toil, but if laced with sugar and accompanied by a favourite snack bar, appetite for the next meal is blunted and all the ills of the saccharine disease made more likely.

Housewives, bamboozled by intensive advertising, are bound to ask, 'Do we not need sugar for energy?' The answer is that the human body will get all the energy it requires from foods which have not been artificially sweetened. During the opening decades of the nineteenth century, sugar consumption was a modest 10 to 12 lb. per person annually, in contrast to today's consumption of approximately 100 lb. This was in the days of Wellington and Nelson when our soldiers and sailors performed feats of physical endurance unsurpassed in modern times. A small annual intake of sugar, say under 15 lb. per person per annum, would allow households to make their own marmalade and jam which, taken in moderate quantities to enhance the taste of whole-wheat bread, would surely do their families no harm. Some commercial jams and marmalades are made without additives other than sugar; but many are coloured by artificial dyes.

2. *Refined white flour.* Try to find bread made from 100 per cent extraction wholewheat; many commercial breads, advertised as 'natural', are made from white flour with varying amounts of added bran. Cookery books abound, giving recipes for bread-making or baking with unrefined flour. My wife makes delicious wholemeal pastry. In appendix II of Mrs Doris Grant's book *Your Daily Food*[2] are excellent simple recipes, including that for the now illustrious 'Grant loaf'.[1]

3. *Processed fats.* Avoid margarines, 'low fat spreads' and processed

1. T. L. Cleave, *Peptic Ulcer* (Bristol, John Wright, 1962)
2. D. Grant, *Your Daily Food* (London, Faber, 1973)

vegetable oils, which, as detailed in chapter 17, are the end-product of complicated industrial manipulation. Use only natural animal fats such as butter and lard; or unprocessed vegetable oil, such as olive oil.

Daily meals

The following menu is my attempt to eat according to the teaching of McCarrison and Cleave.

Breakfast. Muesli or oatmeal porridge. Many commercial breakfast foods are made with varying quantities of added sugar; they should be avoided. Fresh fruit enhances the taste and value of muesli; so does milk, cream and yoghurt according to the taste and inclination of the consumer. Muesli base is now available for those who wish to add their own fruits, nuts and other ingredients.

Oatmeal porridge should be made from plain oatmeal and not from 'porridge oats'; the latter are precooked and have, to me, an unpleasantly slimy consistency. Porridge cooked without salt is horribly insipid; milk and/or cream or top of the milk add to the taste and nutritional value of oatmeal porridge. For families who like a cooked dish to follow, there is, in my opinion, no harm in the traditional course of cooked eggs, bacon, fish or sausages, as long as the frying pan is not used too often. We are lucky to live in an area where butchers still make their own sausages; many of the mass-produced brands taste awful, appear to contain very little meat and are heavily laced with various additives.

Toast made from white bread has so long been part of breakfast that there is often reluctance to change to wholewheat bread or wholewheat rolls. Many bakers now sell genuine wholewheat products; families who know the true value of real food and who bake their own wholewheat bread are unlikely to want to return to white bread even when toasted.

Lunch. Soups, salads, cheese, wholewheat bread, oatcakes and butter, fresh fruits. Glass of whole milk. I do not believe that there is any benefit to health in skimmed milk.

Supper. Main dish of eggs, meat, poultry, fish or game. Vegetables, freshly cooked or as salads. Potatoes. Herbs are better flavouring agents than commercial sauces. Fruit salad, including dried fruits, when available. Cooks who wish to make exotic desserts with the minimum of added sugar will find help in the book departments of health food shops, especially Mrs Libby Day's book, *A Taste of Health*.[3, 4]

Questions

The following questions invariably arise when a dietary regime on the above lines is advocated:

Cost and custom. How can a mother, maybe a single parent with a low income, brought up in one of our huge cities, conditioned since birth to getting all her food precooked, in cans or packages, possibly change her dietary habits? I am well aware that to a considerable proportion, maybe the majority, of our population meals such as I have detailed might at first be unacceptable, and that to some, the advice to grow your own vegetables would be almost beyond comprehension. But the complaint that a health-giving diet is too expensive is not sustained by detailed costings published by Mrs Maisie Steven,[5] author of *The Good Scots Diet*.[6] Mrs Steven, with wide experience as community nutritionist, hospital dietician and college lecturer, has priced meals for one day (at 1983 values) as follows: conventional processed foods, including white bread, processed breakfast food, mince and potatoes, apple tarts, sweet biscuits, etc.: £2.36. Health-giving food including fresh fruits and vegetables, bacon and egg pie, cheese, wholewheat bread and oatcakes: £1.11. The 'processed' meal is more than double the price of the recommended one.

At a time of high unemployment and poverty, family health and solvency could be greatly enhanced by the yields of fruits and vegetables from a family allotment. In most of our cities there is no lack of available land for this purpose; only will and know-how are lacking. Cultivating a patch of land is maybe not everyone's cup of tea, but would not this endeavour give purpose to the lives of men unable so far to find employment?

But how can I wean my baby? Harassed mothers, as they start to wean their babies from breast or bottle, may well greet with dismay advice to avoid canned infant foods. Widespread dependence on these canned products was recently revealed by public expressions of panic and

3. Libby Day, *A Taste for Health* (London, Foulsham, 1985)
4. Jane Horsely, *Sugar Free Cook Book* (Bridport, Prism Press, 1983)
5. Maisie Stevens, 'A better diet for Scotland', *Nutrition and Health*, vol. 2, no. 22 (1983)
6. Maisie Stevens, *The Good Scots Diet* (Aberdeen University Press, 1986)

emergency when, because of a scare of criminal contamination, certain brands of canned baby foods had to be withdrawn. To many households it seemed that no other way existed for feeding infants.

Many excellent, inexpensive hand-operated appliances are available, which easily and quickly convert solid foods to purees. Varied fresh foods can in this way be offered to weaned infants who will thus be spared the risks of consuming artificial sweeteners, dyes and other additives.

My children crave sweets. Are children to be denied sweets, soft drinks, commercial ice cream and so forth? If a sugar tax rationed these worthless products (they are not foods), more children would turn to fruit to satisfy their craving for sweetness; but what a political storm would blow! And how the sugar trade would fan the fires of protest! There must be an evolutionary explanation for the strength of the human desire for sweetness in foods; my guess is the fact that human beings, unlike almost all mammals, are unable to manufacture vitamin C in their own bodies from other foodstuffs. Without this vitamin (see chapter 11) life is not possible. It was therefore essential that our ancestors who, for millions of years, got their food by hunting and gathering, should search for vitamin-rich sweet-tasting foods and roots in order to balance savoury tasting meats. A vast network of industries now caters for our desire for sweetness. From infancy our children are conditioned to the taste of an artificially sweetened nourishment.

In the face of mass advertising and of confectionery displays everywhere, conscientious parents are faced with an uphill task. School tuck shops do not help, nor do indulgent relatives. Sweets taken immediately after meals are probably less harmful than when eaten between meals, and some families succeed in sticking to this rule. Home-made ice cream tastes infinitely better than the commercial product. Less difficulty may be experienced in guiding children to avoid artificially sweetened and artificially coloured soft drinks, by offering them unadulterated (but more expensive) fruit juice.

Is childhood hyperactivity a myth? Increasing evidence confirms the experience of some families that in a minority of children intolerance to certain foods or food additives causes disturbed behaviour, sometimes exploding as severe mental illness. As usual, disagreement reigns in the medical profession about the role of food intolerance or allergy in causing mental symptoms. Psychologists tend to emphasise how some families, in order to escape from the label of emotional instability,

211

latch on to supposed food intolerance as the cause of their psychological difficulties; these professional critics quote numerous cases in which double-blind testing fails to demonstrate adverse symptoms as long as the identity of the supposedly harmful food is disguised. Their findings suggest that families cling to the more comforting diagnosis of food allergy; they are merely 'allergic' to the possibility of symptoms being psychological in origin.

Some consultant paediatricians condemn 'alarmist books, uncritical coverage by the media, and misguided advice by health professions'[7] for encouraging parents to blame food rather than facing other causes of misbehaviour in their offspring; but there is nothing alarmist in Dr Richard Mackarness's account of his work in the psychiatric department of Park Prewett Hospital, Basingstoke,[8] nor in the careful studies of Dr Ian Menzies, Consultant Child Psychiatrist, Tayside Health Board, Dundee.[9] The gratitude of parents and of patients, rescued from utmost misery by simple dietary change or the removal of a harmful environmental agent, is proof of the importance of this subject; it is, however, one of complexity. The manifestations of food intolerance or allergy arise from the interaction of various 'stresses' on the human body; these include the stresses induced by specific foods, food additives and possibly unknown qualities in foods grown with chemicals. The effects of these physical agents can be worsened by psychological stresses, especially fatigue; the exact mechanism may be very difficult to unravel, but what has already been discovered gives a glimpse of a vast new territory of cause and effect which may lead us to understand the origins of hitherto baffling mental diseases.[10]

I used to think that the claims of the pioneers of the new 'environmental medicine' were greatly exaggerated, but repeated discussion with Drs Mackarness and Menzies and experience in practice have convinced me that intolerance to certain foods and food additives is real and serious. In any case, advice to avoid, as far as possible, artificially dyed and sweetened confectionery and soft drinks is in keeping with the philosophy of Cleave and McCarrison.

What about honey? Production of honey on a commercial scale would be impossible without the use of sugar for feeding bees and of modern equipment to protect the beekeeper; thus wild honey in ancient times

7. Anne Wiltshire, 'Hyperactive children, hysterical parents', *Independent*, 13 February 1990
8. R. Mackarness, *Chemical Victims* (London, Pan Books, 1980)
9. Ian Menzies, 'Diet and troubled children', *Health at School*, vol. 1, 1986, pp. 161–2
10. A. Gettis, 'Food sensitivities and psychological disturbance, a review', *Nutrition and Health*, vol. 6, no. 3. (1989), pp. 135–46

was difficult to collect and was prized as a luxury. Cleave believed that honey, like refined sugar, if taken in large quantities would cause those diseases associated with overconsumption (see chapter 15). He reminded us of Proverbs 25, verse 27: 'It is not good to eat too much honey'. The same chapter of Proverbs also states (verse 16): 'Hast thou found honey? Eat so much as is sufficient for thee, lest thou be filled therewith and vomit'. So eat honey sparingly!

Is deep freezing harmful? Freezing is probably the least harmful way of preserving selected foods; but freezing should serve as a back-up to, not a substitute for, fresh food; freezers use fossil-fuel energy and are not necessary for the provision of fresh vegetables, even during a Scottish winter (see chapter 24).

Is irradiated food safe? No scientist knows the full extent of the health-giving qualities which reside in 'live' fruits and vegetables. By 'live', I mean the capacity of root vegetables to sprout and of the seeds of fruits or vegetables to germinate. Irradiation kills this capacity and gives a bogus appearance of freshness. Irradiated foods should be avoided.

Should meat be avoided? Meat and meat products, kidney, liver, etc., are valuable, and for most consumers, appetising foods; in countries like Scotland, mountainous marginal lands will provide no other food in quantity. In prehistoric times, the hill tribes of the north lived mostly on the meat and milk from their cattle;[11] Julius Caesar noted that most of the inland Britons 'did not sow corn but lived on milk and meat'.[12] The fat in meat enhances its flavour, but the fashion for low-fat cuts has recently substituted lean, relatively tasteless meat for the far tastier traditional Aberdeen Angus.

In arable lands, however, meat production from cattle is an inefficient way of converting soil fertility to food. McCarrison's Hunzas had to conserve their lands with great care; they consumed meat about once a week and relied on milk and eggs for animal protein.

Muscle meat is a good source of zinc, iron and B vitamins, but a poor source of vitamins C and A. Peoples having no access to fruits or vegetables correct these deficiencies by eating vitamin-rich animal organs – kidneys, liver, bone marrow, blood, and so on; hence the

11. W. Gauld, 'Native and Roman in Glenalmond', *Journal of Perthshire Society for Natural Science* (1987) vol. 15, pp. 31–9
12. *Ibid*

value of the Scottish haggis made from the liver, heart and lungs of a sheep.

Are aluminium pots harmful? It is not known if the use of aluminium cooking vessels contributes to the cause of Alzheimer's disease (or 'pre-senile dementia'). The role of aluminium in this disease remains obscure – another area of uncertainty, confusion and guesswork.

Is salt bad for us? Excessive amounts of salt, eaten by people overdependent on food salted for preservation, may well be harmful, but there is no evidence that salt, used moderately as a flavouring agent, will do us any harm. The theory that salt causes high blood pressure in advanced nations is controversial.

What about working mothers? We cannot escape this question; fresh food for family meals means careful shopping and daily toil in the kitchen, toil which is unending and exhausting and which cannot be done by a mother engaged in full-time work away from home. I will incur the wrath of militant feminists in suggesting that there can be no more worthwhile, creative job than providing health-giving meals for a growing family. Many husbands for too long may well have selfishly sloped off to the pub or golf course when they should have been supporting their wives in the kitchen. Women have every right before marriage to seek qualifications and careers in business or profession, but the priority of providing sound nutrition for growing children imposes constraints which cannot be avoided. These constraints need not bar a mother from a career outside her home once her children are grown; indeed a mature mother will be a far better shopkeeper, business or professional woman.

Supporting societies

Parents concerned for the health of their families, and farmers considering a switch to organic production, can be greatly helped by various organisations established in the last fifty years. There are now so many that I will not attempt to list them all, but will briefly discuss the societies of which I have some knowledge.

The Soil Association. Founded immediately after World War II, it owed its conception and birth to the late Lady Eve Balfour, who determined

Appendix 1

to explore the relationship between soil fertility and health. (See chapter 24 on the founding of the Soil Association.)

Unfortunately, the Association's Council could not agree on the priority for basic research, which Lady Eve believed should be foremost among the Society's objectives. Perhaps it was inevitable that the mounting expense of the Haughley experiment (research based on three self-contained side-by-side farms at Haughley in Suffolk) made impossible its survival under a relatively small, and financially poor, independent association.[13]

Today the Soil Association continues the campaign for organic farming; it runs the symbol scheme, designed to protect us from traders who might cash in on the higher prices commanded by organic produce, and publishes a quarterly journal, *The Living Earth*. The Association has recently launched a campaign to achieve 20 per cent of British farm production by organic methods by the end of the century.

Two other organisations, allied to the Soil Association, are giving a lead in the growing and marketing of organic produce; they are British Organic Farmers (BOF) and Organic Growers Association (OGA). Information on these and on the Soil Association is available at 86–88 Colston Street, Bristol, Avon BS1 5BB.

Elm Farm Research Centre. An organic advisory service has now been established as an educational charity at Elm Farm Research Centre, near Newbury in Berkshire, under the direction of Lawrence Woodward. Here practical advice including advisory visits to farms is available to farmers who wish to convert to organic methods. The address is Organic Advisory Service, Elm Farm Research Centre, Hampstead Marshall, near Newbury, Berkshire RG15 0HR.

The Henry Doubleday Research Association (HDRA). Founded in 1954 and named after Henry Doubleday (1813–1902), son of a prosperous Quaker, who championed the plant Russian comfrey as a prodigious cropper (100 to 120 tons to the acre) and the source of valuable nutrients for livestock. Comfrey (*Symphytum asperrimum*) was prized in antiquity as a healing agent. Henry Doubleday spent much of his life researching its quality; he believed that the plant might be the answer to the needs of a hungry world. (Unfortunately, all his research papers were destroyed, so no one knows what he discovered.) The success of the association named after him is due, as was the success of the

13. E. Balfour, *The Living Soil* (London, Faber, 1975)

215

Soil Association, to the drive and ability of one person, in this instance the late Lawrence Hills, who has done for the future of gardening what Lady Eve did for farming.

Lawrence Hills (1911–1990), from childhood possessed of a burning curiosity in natural science, triumphed in spite of terrible adversity. His growing years were punctuated by devastating episodes of coeliac disease in the days when the very simple cause of that condition was not understood. The offending substance, gluten, a protein of wheat and other cereals, reacts with intestinal lining and prevents normal absorption of food; symptoms of indigestion, diarrhoea, failure to thrive, anaemia and weakness usually start in infancy; health is restored when foods containing cereal gluten are avoided. In spite of this affliction Lawrence worked long and hard in various horticultural institutions and acquired a formidable reserve of experience as a practical grower. He had a flair as an author on horticultural subjects, published a book on alpines and was a prolific contributor as a horticultural correspondent.[14]

Convinced of the importance of the research on Russian comfrey, started by Henry Doubleday, Lawrence determined to continue the work by setting up a research plot in which other aspects of organic growing could also be explored. He did so in 1953 when, with his parents, he bought a house and rented a neighbouring plot at Braintree in Essex. The Hills received no government grant, no massive financial backing; but Lawrence's skills as a communicator and writer attracted increasing interest in and membership of the Association. Under his direction, a growing network of gardeners participated in trials in their own gardens of the techniques of organic growing. A series of successful books and pamphlets dealing with all aspects of gardening flowed from Lawrence's pen.

In a few years, the HDRA achieved recognition as a charity devoted to research and education in organic gardening and farming. In the 1960s Lawrence's health was fully restored when he married Cherry (Hilda Brooke), physiotherapist and dietician. She prescribed his gluten-free diet. Gone for ever were the coeliac episodes. In 1984 Allan Gear and his wife Jackie were enrolled as HDRA managers and in 1985, having sold the Braintree properties, the Association moved to a much larger and more easily accessible site at Ryton, near Coventry. With a membership of some 17,000 the HDRA is the largest organic growers' association in the world.

---

14. L. Hills, *Fighting Like the Flowers* (Bideford, Green Books, 1989)

For any gardener who has interest in growing for the kitchen, I urge a visit to the demonstration gardens at Ryton; the centre includes a shop and pleasant restaurant. The outstanding value of the HDRA is its devotion to practice as well as to theory. The shop at Ryton includes a large collection of organic literature, but reading is greatly enhanced by seeing, and the garden shows organic methods in action. The HDRA publishes a quarterly newsletter, and markets an extensive range of seeds, plants and gardening aids. The address is HDRA, National Centre for Organic Gardening, Ryton-on-Dunsmore, Coventry CV8 1LG.

The McCarrison Society. At a Soil Association weekend conference, held at Attingham Park, near Shrewsbury, in 1965, a small group of members, qualified doctors or dentists, decided to form a society devoted to the study of nutrition and health, membership to be limited to applicants holding a degree in medicine, dentistry or veterinary science. After a series of preliminary meetings and discussions arranged by the late Dr James Mount, the McCarrison Society was established in 1966. The late Dr Innes Pearce, well known for her work as the co-founder of the Peckham Pioneer Health Centre, gave valuable advice. We hoped to enrol practising doctors, dentists and vets and to hasten the understanding of prevention by sound nutrition as advocated by McCarrison.

But professionals did not seem eager to join, and membership increased but slowly. A number of successful and well-attended summer conferences were held in the 1970s at Oxford thanks to the enthusiasm and skilful management of the then secretary, Dr Barbara Latto, and the faithful treasurer, dental surgeon Ken Rose. In 1982 Dr Andrew Strigner, the then chairman of the society, cooperated with Dr Hugh Sinclair of Oxford in arranging anew publication of McCarrison's *Nutrition and Health*, originally published by Faber. Another chairman, Dr Kenneth Barlow, in association with A. B. Academic Publishers launched an international journal, *Nutrition and Health*, which continues under the editorship of Dr Edward Kirby. In 1976 membership was extended to applicants with a qualification in dietetics or allied sciences. A Scottish and a North England group have more recently been established. The present chairman is Professor Michael Crawford, The Institute of Brain Chemistry and Nutrition, Queen Elizabeth Hospital for Children, Hackney Road, London E2 8PS, tel. 071–739 8422. President, Professor David Morley, Institute of Child Health, London University, Secretary, Richard Longhurst, Centre for International Child Health, London University. The Scottish Chairman is Dr Cedric Devoil, 5 Albert Street, Arbroath, Tayside, tel. 0241 72614. Scottish Secretary is Tom Smith, Loanhead, Kingskettle, Fife KY7 PJ.

Foresight. This is a charity devoted to educating parents on the valuable role of sound nutrition in preventing morbidity associated with pregnancy. Foresight has produced pamphlets emphasising the importance of educating parents before conception in order to ensure a trouble-free pregnancy and a healthy baby. One of their booklets is a valuable guide to shoppers for identifying food additives according to their E code on container labels. Information from Mrs Peter Barnes, Foresight, The Old Vicarage, Church Lane, Witley, Surrey, GU8 5PN.

The National Childbirth Trust. Has already been mentioned in chapter 3. Enquiries to Alexandra House, Oldham Terrace, London W3 6NH, tel. 081–992 8637.

APPENDIX 2

Advice to Government

In this second appendix, I venture to advise measures which only governments can take. These should be as few as possible. We are already overgoverned, and the history of government intervention in land use for food production in peacetime does not inspire confidence. Governments should not tell us what we must eat or drink, but the following tax and fiscal changes would, in my opinion, help those who search for health. I am well aware that my suggestions will be met on all sides by ridicule and scorn as being hopelessly impracticable. If implemented, they would lead to widespread changes in the fertiliser and food processing industry and in farming; some repopulation of the countryside would have to follow expansion of organic farming. Such changes would provoke intense political opposition; but having witnessed in my lifetime the astonishing changes in the climate of opinion in matters pertaining to human health, I know how swiftly beliefs, which today are rejected as nonsense, can tomorrow become accepted wisdom.

In democracies, where freedom of speech yet endures, official attitudes can still be changed by public opinion. For years the organic movement was subjected to official scorn; that it has survived and has apparently now earned the blessing of the minister of agriculture is due to the efforts, not of government nor of colleges of agriculture, but of humble individuals and independent societies, who received no financial backing from official quarters.

The record of official policies in the prevention of modern diseases is lamentable. The publication of McCarrison's research and recommendations in 1936 were ignored by the government, by its official advisers and by the medical profession; forty years later, in 1976, the role of sound nutrition in prevention was still not recognised. In that year a government booklet *Prevention and Health: Everybody's Business*[1] devoted one brief complacent paragraph to nutrition. Only now, when the prevalence and staggering costs of modern disease have brought our country near to bankruptcy, is the government belatedly giving priority to prevention.

I have nine points to urge upon the government:

1. Sugar tax. A substantial tax on refined sugar is perfectly logical. Even those who neglect or deride the teaching of Cleave, accept that, in the quantities in which it is being consumed in the UK today, refined sugar is the main cause of dental decay and contributes to the causes of obesity. Both of these common diseases cost the taxpayers enormous sums of money; why should those who eat and produce sugar not help to pay its costs? If my calculations are correct a tax of 2p per pound of sugar would yield over £100 million, assuming that the present per caput consumption is 100lb per annum.

Forecasting scientific developments is notoriously difficult; but it is certain that fossil fuels will one day be exhausted. Fuel from plants, especially sugar cane, may become a valuable, sustainable means of powering internal combustion engines. Such fuel would, I suppose, be very expensive and would be exempt from the sugar tax.

2. White flour tax. The same argument applies in favour of a tax on highly refined flour and on polished rice. Fibre-depleted foods, as explained in earlier chapters, cause constipation and the complications of that distressing condition. Again the cost in expenditure of public money and in human disability is enormous. Again those who choose to produce and to eat these foods should contribute to the costs.

Ideally, our daily bread should come from freshly ground, organically-grown wholewheat flour; such idealism would require a decentralised milling industry to supply freshly ground flour to local bakeries in every township, so that wholewheat bread could be marketed at a lower price than white.

3. Food additives. All synthetic dyes at present used to colour food and drink should be banned. As explained in chapter 10, many of these are derived from petrochemicals.

4. Food labelling. The 'E' coding system should be replaced by full

---

1. *Prevention and Health: Everybody's Business* (London, HMSO, 1976)

lists of all additives, grouped as to their function and written in letters large enough easily to be read. Preservatives are necessary additions to mass-produced convenience foods; but consumers have every right to know exactly what they are eating. Similar strict laws should apply to commercial cattle feed. Farmers have a right to know exactly what their beasts are eating.

5. Agriculture and fisheries. The European Common Agricultural Policy – an expensive, bureaucratic, corrupt, food-destroying disaster[2] – must be scrapped. Should not each European country be responsible for the way in which it uses its own land and for the preservation of its own fish stocks? Within a coastal limit of twelve miles or more sovereign nations should have absolute right to decide who should be permitted to fish in their waters and the right to use their navies to protect those waters. Urgent action is required to preserve the life of coastal seabeds which are rapidly being destroyed by modern trawling techniques.

A substantial tax should be levied on all soluble nitrogenous fertilisers, which depress and disrupt the mechanisms of natural fertility and pollute our drinking water. The costs of nitrate pollution are considerable and should be met by producers and users. The following measures might help farmers who wish to 'go organic':

i. A complete ban on the use of certain highly toxic pesticides. On present evidence, I would suggest all chlorinated hydrocarbons and all organophosphates. A similar ban on toxic herbicides.

ii. Diversion of some of the cash raised by the above taxes to research and development of organic methods and to helping organisations like the Soil Association and the HDRA, which already run advisory services for the benefit of organic farmers and gardeners.

iii. Priority should be given to research on recycling human wastes including sewage. In Germany, a commercially successful scheme for converting household wastes into good quality compost has already been established under the guidance of the Department of Agriculture of the University of Kassel.[3] If such schemes are to include human excrement a way must be found for disposing of toxic industrial wastes without contaminating sewage, so that the latter is made fit

2. R. Cottrell, *The Sacred Cow* (London, Grafton Books, 1987)
3. H. Vogtmann, Department of Agriculture, University of Kassel, personal communication to the author, 1986

for incorporation in municipal composts. The expense would be considerable but we cannot indefinitely go on dumping our sewage in our estuaries and increasingly fouling seas and beaches. Animal dung is one of nature's essential ingredients in the working of the law of return which governs soil fertility. Human excrement is still used as an important fertiliser in many parts of the world. Is it beyond our wit, in industrial nations, safely to channel our wastes in order to enhance soil fertility? As water becomes increasingly scarce and expensive, a dry toilet designed to yield 1 cwt. per annum of a high-potash compost from a family of three adults is surely worth developing; such a device, invented in Sweden, is amusingly described by the late Lawrence Hills in his recently published autobiography.[4] If such a toilet can really be safely used, it would save millions of gallons of water and would certainly solve the problem of contamination of sewage by industrial wastes.

6. Allotments.   The provision of land for householders who wish to grow their own vegetables, fruits and flowers should be an essential part of all local authority planning. Community education departments should be encouraged to give high priority to the expansion of allotments.

7. Education and Advertising.   Something must be done to protect the public from advertisements masquerading as nutritional science. For many years the law has forbidden the sale of medicines advertised as cures for cancer or tuberculosis; the same reasoning should apply to foods advertised as promoting health. The following measures are now necessary:

i. Any scientist who writes, for publication, a paper or book on the subject of nutrition and health and who does not reveal the fact that he has received financial help from or is in the regular pay of a commercial enterprise, may be prosecuted.

ii. The distribution of educational material on nutrition and health by food manufacturers to schools, colleges or other educational establishments should be made illegal. I do not know how the editors of farming journals can be protected from the financial power of agrichemical advertisers who have used the threat of withdrawal of advertising revenue in order to influence editorial policy; but could

---

4. L. Hills, *Fighting like the Flowers* (Bridford, Green Books, 1989), pp. 221–5

not sensible legislation prevent multinationals peddling PR material (usually free) disguised as an editorial?[5]

iii. In medical schools more time must be allocated to studies on ecology and on prevention by sound nutrition. The education of children should include, from an early age, teaching on the value of health-giving food.

iv. Teachers of home economics in schools and colleges should be trained to understand the importance of nutrition in human health; the foods served in many of these establishments show a woeful lack of understanding of what constitutes a health-giving meal!

8. Forestry. The nurture and harvesting of trees for timber, food, shelter, soil and climate conservation is a top priority in land use. I cannot dwell on this subject but wish to join those who protest at the blanket of conifer monoculture now covering so many of our Scottish hills. Financial manipulation by tax or subsidy should surely encourage the revival of native hard woods and their use as shelter belt or for furniture and building.

9. Ministry of Land Use and Health. The above measures might be better coordinated if the Ministries of Food, Agriculture and Fisheries and the Ministry of Health were to be abolished and replaced by a single ministry of Land Use and Health. This suggestion was made in 1972 by the late Professor Lindsay Robb when he said:

> This (the new Ministry of Land Use and Health) would focus attention simultaneously on the most fundamental of human and soil problems and provide the most effective organisation for contributing to human health through its basic source – a fertile soil.

Professor Robb, an authority on soil conservation and agriculture, was successively a practical farmer, grassland advisor to ICI, a professor of agriculture in South Africa and finally an adviser to the FAO. His warnings given in the 1950s of starvation, soil erosion and drought in Africa appear to have been remarkably accurate.

The existing Health Service would be renamed the National *Medical Service*. The ending of the Orwellian use of the word 'health' in relation to medical care (when what is meant is 'disease') might remind the

---

5. G. Harvey, 'Calling the tune?' *New Farmer and Grower*, no. 27 (1990), pp. 12, 13
6. R. L. Robb, 'Man and soil, mountain top to city pavement', Sanderson Wells Lecture (1957) printed in *Journal of the Soil Association*, vol. 17, no. 2 (1972)

thoughtless that our health depends not on the activities of doctors and their professional helpers, however expert they are in repairing our infirmities, but on the soundness of our diet. A ministry of Land Use and Health would have to review the present laissez-faire policy on the buying and selling of land; land is surely too precious a possession to be left at the mercy of international financiers or even to wealthy citizens of other countries.

Index

AIDS and the permissive society 180
Aberfeldy Water Mill 129
alcohol 77
allergy 212
appendicitis and abscess
    formation 130; and bowel
    infection 130; and disease
    clustering 136; history in
    Edinburgh Royal Infirmary 131;
    King Edward VII 134; and
    plumbing technology 136; and
    stress factors 117–8
arteriosclerosis in diabetes 109; and
    saturated fats 146
asthma, recent increase 82
auto-immune disease 125

BSE 196
Balfour, Lady Eve and ecology 185;
    Haughley Experiment 185; *The
    Living Soil* 185
Barfield, A. 150
Bell, Joseph 134
birth defects in Scotland 97; and
    vitamin deficiency 97
blood glucose, control of 108
Boyd-Orr, Lord 149
Bougie landing 169
breast-feeding, delivery routine 38;

modern trends 74; and social
    class 77
Burkett, Mr D. 61

COMA report on dietary
    sugars 163–4
Cajanus Journal 162
Cameron, Jessie, Matron, Aberfeldy
    Cottage Hospital 31
Campbell, Dr G. D. 149
cancer and agri-chemicals 81, 84,
    192–3; in Asian
    republics 119–200; colonic 79;
    gastro-intestinal 73; in
    Scotland 81; and tobacco 81
carbohydrates, digestion and
    metabolism 107; over-
    consumption 106
Caribbean, dietary intakes 161–3
Carson, Rachael 192
Carstairs, Prof. M. 179
Cheshire Medical Testament 186
childbed fever 93
childbirth in rural practice 31
chloroform in rural obstetrics 32
cholesterol, blood levels and egg
    consumption 148; and cancer 85;
    and coronary heart disease 146;
    lowering and gallstones 157;
    National Education program,

USA 158; and violence 159;
WHO study 156
Cleave, T. L. awards 1979 63; and
evolution 65, 106; and varicose
veins 60
Clofibrate 156
Common Agricultural Policy 188;
and waste 201–02
compost for vegetable plots 46
constipation and varicose veins 60
consumer groups and organic
farming 202
coronary thrombosis in the
Caribbean 161; in Cuba 164; and
disease clustering 144; and
exercise 140; and genetic
factors 143; in Harrow and
Brent 150; history of 143; in
Korean War, American
soldiers 157; and sugar
consumption 165; and tobacco
smoking 145; in USA 157, 160; and
vegetable oils 149

Dedichen, Dr Jens 155
dental caries and bone
structure 35–6
depopulation, rural 21, 190
diabetes, complications 109; in
Dominica 162; increasing
evidence 112; incubation
period 136; in Natal Indians 149;
and stress 118
Dick-Read, Dr Grantley 32
diverticular disease, prevention 72
Doll, Sir Richard 61, 63
Dunn, Dr Peter M. 37
duodenal ulcer, history 115; and
polished rice consumption 115;
and protein stripping 116; and
stress 117

Elm Farm Research Centre 215
exercise 139–40

family, as biological unit 182
farming, recent changes 21

fatigue, in battle 44; in general
practice 44
fats, dietary, advertising 147;
consumption in Europe in
relation to coronary
thrombosis 150–1; energy
from 163; WHO publication 150
Fergusson, Dr Somerled 140
fertiliser, chemical, addictive
effect 187–8; and use of
ammonium nitrate 190–1; and
cancer 83, 84, 191; and
pollution 199; and Scottish
colleges of agriculture 190; and
selenium deficiency 84, 191; and
trace element deficiency 84
fibre, dietary, transit times 69
First Army in Africa 169
flour milling, mineral loss 60
fluoride, a waste product 196–197;
Court of Session case 197–8;
naturally occurring in hard
water 197; and Royal College of
Physicians' Report 197–8
folic acid in pregnancy 97
food additives 220; allergy and
rheumatism 121
Food Combining for Health and
rheumatism 120
Franconfonte village, battle 171
Freud, Sigmund 116; and
Christianity 179
Furth, Dr Anna 111

gardening, market 46; UNICEF/
WHO Report 200; vegetable
yields 188
Gilchrist, Dr Rae 142–3
Glubb, Sir John 177–8
glycation, of protein 110–1
Grant, Mrs Doris, and food
combining 120

Haemolytic streptococcus, and
rheumatic disease 127
Hahnemann, Dr S. C. F. 126
Hay, Dr and food combining 121
Henderson, Dr J. 143

Index

Henry Doubleday Research Association 215–7
Highland Division (51st) 170–6
Highlands and Islands Medical Service 23
homeopathy 125–7
Howard, Sir Albert 185
humus, and soil fertility 185
Hunzas 115, 213; and dietary regime 84
hyperactive children 211, 212
hyperinsulinism 109–10
hypoglycaemic coma 109

Imperial decline through history 177–8; and soil erosion 184
industrial revolution, cheap food policy 195–6; population imbalance 195
infant mortality, in Asian republics 200
insulin 108

Jamesfield Farm 189
Japan, sugar consumption 153
Joice, Jean, and food combining 120–121

labour, induction of 33
Lamb, Col. G. B. M. 172
Line, Dr James 89
longevity in Hunzas 53; in rural Scotland 70
Lutz, Dr Wolfgang 147

magnesium deficiency in pregnancy 34–5
margarine, expanding consumption 146; manufacturing process 152
Marx, Karl, and Christianity 179, 198; and the Russian Revolution 198
Masai tribe and fat consumption 148
McCarrison, Sir Robert, and appendicitis 135–6; classic rat-feeding experiments 181:

society 217
Mackarness, Dr Richard 212
McKenzie, Sir James, history of coronary thrombosis 135
Medical Research Council and coronary heart disease 160–1; survey on sugar consumption 165
Mediterranean diet and coronary thrombosis 152–3
Menzies, Dr Ian 212
migraine 119–120
milk products, in antiquity 147–8; in Scottish Highlands 151
Millar, Ian 189
Mills, Sir John 121
Montgomery, Captain RAMC 171
Moore, Thomas 158
mycorrhizal association 187–8

Natal Indians, incidence of diabetes and coronary thrombosis 149–50
National Health Insurance Act 1911 186
Natural Childbirth 32; Association 33; delivery position 37
nitrates and water pollution 188
Noble, Major Tony 172
nutrition in pregnancy 34–5

oatmeal 209
Odent, Dr Michael 39
olive oil 152
organic food and cancer 83; growing and natural law 187, 196; and rural depopulation 190

Painter, Dr N. S. 61, 72
palm oil 152
Passmore, Dr R. 115
Pauling, Dr L. 91
Pearce, Dr Innes 185, 217
Peckham Experiment, the 185
permissive society 179; and abortion 180
pesticides and cancer in USA 192–3; in farming 193; in the Third World 194

227

Index

Picton, Dr Lionel 186
pollution, in Aral Sea 199; and UNICEF/WHO report 199–200
polymyalgia rheumatica 125
polyunsaturated fats 146
Pottinger, Dr F. 185
Price, Weston 35, 185
pudendal block anaesthesia 32
psychoanalysis and modern diseases 116–7
psychosomatic medicine 116–7
puberty, earlier onset 180; and nutrition 181

Reith Lecture, 1962 179
relaxation in childbirth 32
rheumatism, and food combining 120–2; possible causes 123–4
Rousseau, Jean-Jacques 117
Royal College of GPs and nutrition education 187

saccharine disease, the 63
Samburu Tribe and fat consumption 148
saturated fats 146
scarlet fever 138
Schaeffer, Dr Otto 110
science and religion 182–3
Scotland, dietary habits 75–77
Scott-Park, J. 190–1
Scott-Williamson, Dr 185
Scottish farmers and dietary fat controversy 161–2
Scottish Ski Club 44–5
scurvy 89
selenium deficiency 191; and cancer 84
Semmelweiss, Dr Ignaz 93
serotonin, and human behaviour 159–60
sex before marriage 179; and Samoans 179
sex education in Sweden 180
Sferro Hills, battle of 173–6
Short, Dr Rendle 131–2
Sicily landing 170

Sinclair, Dr Hugh 81
Sinclair, Sir John 70
Smith, Revd Coty 171
social class and dietary habits 35; and childbirth 34
Soil Association 214–5; foundation of 185
soil erosion 184
soil fertility and artificial chemicals 187–8; on an organic farm 189; and earth worms 185
Solzhenitsyn, A. 199
Sorel-Cameron, Col. 171
St Mary's Hospital, cholesterol-lowering failure 155–6
Steiner, Rudolf 126
steroids and rheumatic disease 125
Steven, Maisie 70
Stockdale, T. 190
Stott, Dr Halley 48
sugar, age of puberty 181; consumption and human behaviour 181; consumption in Mediterranean 152–3; consumption in UK 208; and duodenal ulcer 208; and expenditure on advertising 146–7
Swanson, Dr C. J. 23; as obstetrician 31
Sweden, health comparison with Scotland 79

Tanner, J. M. 181
temporal arteritis 124–5
Thomson, Alexis 134
Thomson, Dr Anne 49
Thomson, Cameron, and rock dust 194
tobacco smoking and coronary thrombosis 145
Torch, operation, 1942 169
toxaemia of pregnancy 34–5
Treeves, Sir Frederick 134
Trowell, Dr Hugh 118
Tunis, capture of 170
Turner, Dr R. W. D. 161–2
twin, delivery 39–41
typhoid fever 129

Index

USSR and collective farming 199; and Lenin's experiment 198

Valley Trust 48–9
varicose ulcers 53
varicose veins 53; and constipation 60
vitamin C, daily intake 91
vitamin B in pregnancy 35
vitamins, and cancer 83; folic acid in pregnancy 97

WHO European trial 84, 157
Walker, Dr A. R. P. 68
Walker, Prof. James 34
Wimberley, Major-General Douglas 172
Wynn, Arthur and Margaret 81, 99

Yemeni Jews 148
Yudkin, Prof. John 154; and conflict with sugar trade 203

Zieglar, Dr Eugene 110
Zulus, nutritional deficiencies 48–9